TAB

MW01596249

—

INTERMITTENT FASTIN FOR WOMEN OVER 50

The Ultimate Guide To Weight Loss Quickly, Reset
Your Metabolism, Increase Your Energy And
Detox Your Body

By

Stella Waters

policies, processes, or directions contained within is the solitary and utter responsibility of the recipient reader. Under no circumstances will any legal responsibility or blame be held against the publisher for any reparation, damages, or monetary loss due to the information herein, either directly or indirectly.

Respective authors own all copyrights not held by the publisher.

The information herein is offered for informational purposes solely, and is universal as so. The presentation of the information is without contract or any type of guarantee assurance.

The trademarks that are used are without any consent, and the publication of the trademark is without permission or backing by the trademark owner. All trademarks and brands within this book are for clarifying purposes only and are the owned by the owners themselves, not affiliated with this document

CHAPTER 1

UNDERSTANDING INTERMITTENT FASTING

What is intermittent fasting?

We first need to understand the distinction between the fed state and the fasted state to know how intermittent fasting leads to fat loss.

Your body is when it is digesting and absorbing food in the fed state. Typically, when you start eating, the fed state begins and lasts for 3 to 5 hours as your body Absorbs and digest the food you just ate. If you are in the fed state, it's challenging for your body to burn fat because your insulin levels are high.

Your body goes into what is known as the post-absorptive state after that period, which is just a fancy way to say that your body does not process a meal. After your last meal, the post-absorptive state lasts for 8 to 12 hours, when you enter the fasting state. Because your insulin levels are low, it is much easier for your body to burn fat in a fasting state.

Your body can burn fat that has been unavailable during the fed state when you are in the fasting state.

Since we do not enter the fasting state until 12 hours after our last meal, it is uncommon for our bodies to be in this state of fat burning. This is one reason why, without changing what they eat, how much they eat, or how often they exercise, many people who begin intermittent fasting will lose fat. Fasting places your body in a fat-burning state that you seldom do during a normal eating schedule.

EXAMPLES OF DIFFERENT SCHEDULES FOR INTERMITTENT FASTING

There are a few different options for working it into your lifestyle if you're considering giving fasting a shot.

Intermittent Daily Fasting

I follow the Leangain intermittent fasting model most of the time, which uses a 16-hour fast followed by an 8-hour eating period. Martin Berkhan of Leangains.com, the name originated, popularized this intermittent daily fasting model.

When you begin your 8-hour eating period, it does not matter. It's possible to start at 8 a.m. and stop at 4 p.m., Or you're going to begin at 2 p.m. and stop at 10 p.m. Do anything that works for you. I tend to find it works well to eat around 1 p.m. and 8 p.m. because those times allow me to eat with friends and family for lunch and dinner. Breakfast is typically a meal I eat on my own, so it's not a big deal to skip it.

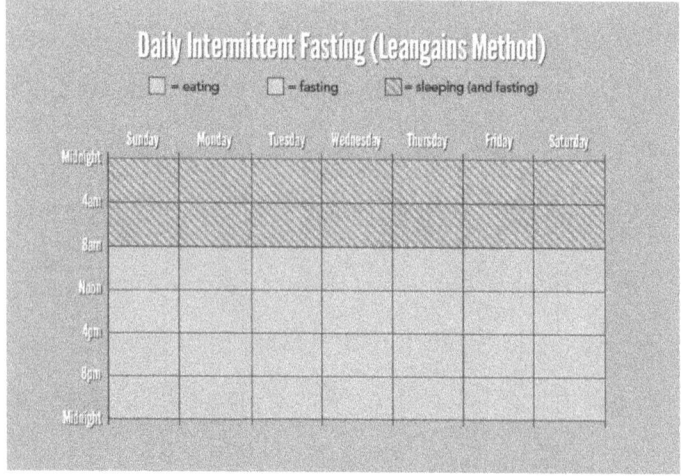

It is very easy to fall into eating on this schedule as intermittent daily fasting is done every day. You probably eat about the same time every day right now without thinking about it. Well, it's the same thing with everyday intermittent fasting. You just learn not to eat at certain hours, which is surprisingly easy.

One potential downside of this schedule is that it becomes harder to get the same amount of calories during the week since you usually take out a meal or two from your day. Put simply, teaching yourself to eat bigger meals daily is difficult. The effect is that many individuals end up losing weight while attempting this form of intermittent fasting. That can depend on your priorities, be a good thing or a bad thing.

This is also a good time to say that I'm not fanatical about my diet, although I've practised intermittent fasting regularly over the last year. 90% of the time, I focus on developing healthy habits that control my actions so that during the other 10%, I can do whatever I feel like. If I go to your house to watch a football match and order a pizza at 11 p.m., guess what? I don't care if it's outside of my feeding time; I eat it.

The Intermittent Weekly Fasting

Doing so once a week or once a month is one of the easiest ways to start intermittent fasting. The occasional rapidity has been shown to contribute to several of the advantages of fasting that we've already spoken about. Still, even if you don't use it to cut calories regularly, fasting also has several other health benefits.

One example of how an intermittent weekly fast could play out is shown in the graphic below.

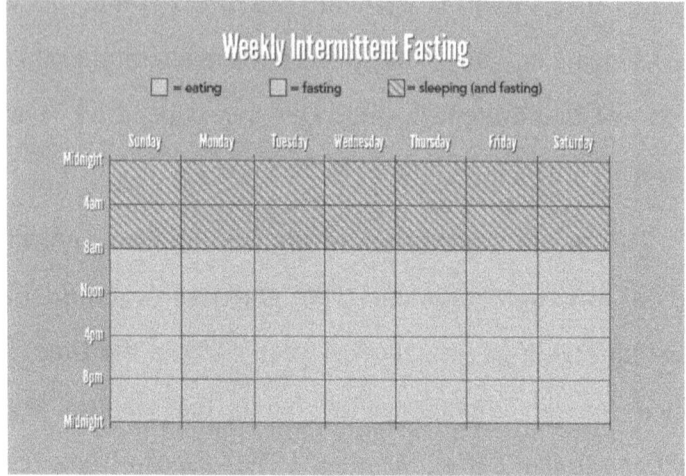

In this case, lunch is your last meal of the day on Monday. Then you fast until Tuesday's lunch. The advantage of this schedule is that you can eat any day of the week while still reaping the fasting benefits for 24 hours. You're less likely to lose weight, too, because you just cut out two meals a week. If you want to bulk up or hang on to weight, this is a great choice.

In the past, I have conducted 24-hour fasts (I just did

one last month), and there are a large variety of combinations and choices to make it work on your timetable. A long day of travel or the day after a major holiday feast, for instance, are also perfect times to put in a 24-hour fast.

Perhaps the greatest advantage of fasting for 24 hours is getting past the mental hurdle of fasting. If you have never fasted before, completing your first one successfully makes you understand that you will not die if you do not eat for a day.

Intermittent Fasting on the Alternative Day

Intermittent fasting on alternate days requires longer fasting times during the week on alternating days.

For instance, you'd eat dinner on Monday night in the graph below and then not eat again until Tuesday evening. You'd eat all day on Wednesday, though, and then resume the 24-hour fasting period again after dinner on Wednesday night. This helps you regularly get long fast periods while consuming at least one meal every day of the week.

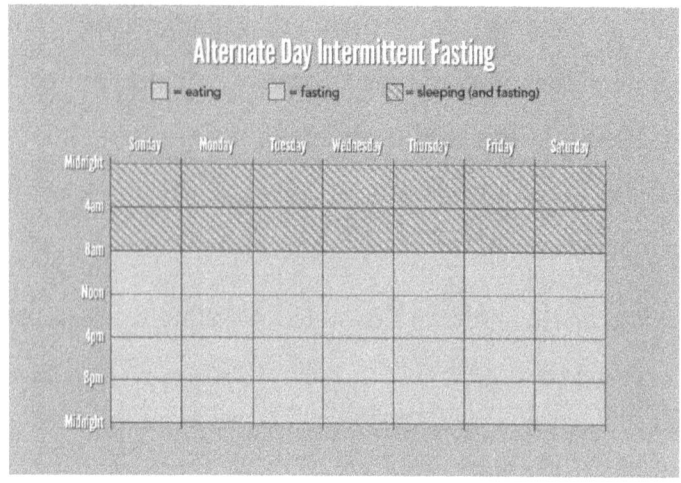

This form of intermittent fasting seems to be mostly used in research studies, but in the real world, from what I have seen, it is not very common. I've never tried fasting on an additional day, and I do not intend to do so.

The advantage of alternate day intermittent fasting is that it gives you a long time in the fasted state than the type of fasting of Leangains. Hypothetically, the advantages of fasting will be improved by this.

I will, however, be concerned with eating enough in practice. Teaching yourself to eat more constantly is one of the tougher aspects of intermittent fasting, based on my experience. You may be able to feast on a meal, but it takes a bit of preparation, a lot of cooking, and consistent eating to learn to do so every day of the week. The result is that most individuals who try to fast intermittently end up losing some weight because, while a few meals are cut out every week, their meals' size remains similar.

This isn't a concern if you're trying to lose weight. And even if you're satisfied with your weight, if you follow your daily fasting or weekly fasting plans, this won't prove to be too much of a problem. However, if you fast on several days a week for 24 hours a day, then it's going to be hard to eat enough of your feast days to make up for that.

As a result, pursuing intermittent daily fasting or a single 24-hour fast once a week or once a month is a safer idea.

Fasting intermittently (IF) can sound technical. But what it implies is to go without feeding for long periods.

Why would anyone want this to be done? The practice will help people lose weight and improve their health, an increasing number of fitness experts argue.

But the sole preserve of diet nerds is hardly intermittent fasting. Every single day we all do some form of it. Except that we're not calling it that. Sleeping, we call it.

That is right. It could characterize the time from your last meal at night until your first meal the next day as a "fasting" interval.

It is as easy as that.

What's the point of fasting?

Though the name may be a recent development, there is nothing new about intermittent fasting.

Either overnight, during longer periods of food shortage, or for religious reasons, humans have often fasted.

Data show that IF can help prolong life, regulate blood glucose, control blood lipids, decrease the risk of cardiovascular disease, manage body weight, help us gain (or maintain) lean mass, decrease the risk of cancer, and more when performed properly.

Now, this research is still in their early stages, so scepticism has plenty of space.

Even so, some of the results look positive. That's so many individuals have chosen to put IF to the test in the fitness world.

I lost body weight and fat, retained lean mass, and managed to do so in a manner that felt manageable. Hey, Performance! Nevertheless, intermittent fasting is not for everybody.

While intermittent fasting has worked for me, it's not a good match for everyone.

Initially, intermittent fasting is not just another way of saying "free ride." It won't help you lose fat or boost your health by skipping meals randomly while eating a diet high in processed foods.

However, there is no "right" way to conduct fasting; there will be a certain amount of attention to nutritional detail in every decent protocol.

To do the job, you have to be prepared. Some would think that IF is too inconvenient or difficult to practice.

And for others, the risks greatly outweigh any possible advantages. In reality, IF may be very dangerous for some individuals. You probably want to know if you fall into that category before missing your next meal.

Intermittently Fasting: Green Light

In my experience, with intermittent fasting, you're most likely to succeed if

- You have a history of monitoring calories and food (e.g., you have "dieted" before).

- You're an accomplished exerciser now,

- You're single, or you have no kids,

- Your partner is incredibly supportive (if you have one),

- Your work allows you to have low-performance times when adapting to a new strategy.

- Well, you're guy,

The first five variables will make it simpler to build the protocols into your lifestyle, while outcomes tend to be influenced by the final condition (being male).

intermittently Fasting: Yellow Light

Meanwhile, you might want to proceed with caution

if you meet the following criteria:

- You're married, or you have kids
- You have jobs that are performance-oriented or client-facing
- In sport/athletics, you play in
- You're a female

Again the first three conditions make it much tougher and can make it impractical for you to obey IF protocols. What's more, trying to go quickly can clash with your sport's performance goals.

As for the last condition, some experimenters say that for women, sleeplessness, anxiety, irregular cycles, and other signs of hormone dysregulation are caused by fasting.

In fact, in the stricter types of intermittent fasting, women seem to do worse than men do. So if you're a woman and want to try fasting, I suggest starting with a relaxed approach.

Intermittently Fasting: Red Light

Finally, some individuals just shouldn't bother at all

with intermittent fasting. Don't try this one if:

- You get pregnant

- You have a history of consuming disordered foods,

- You're under chronic stress

- You're not sleeping well,

- You are new to eating and exercise,

If you're new to exercise and diet, intermittent fasting might look like a weight-loss magic bullet. But before you start playing with fasts, you would be much better to fix any dietary deficiencies. Make sure you first start from a strong nutritional base.

Pregnant women have extra energy requirements, so now is not the time to fast if you start a family.

Ditto if you are under and/or not sleeping under chronic stress. Your body needs nurturing, not extra stress.

And if you've suffered in the past with disordered eating, you probably understand that a fasting regimen could take you down a path that could cause additional issues for you. Why mess with wellbeing? In other ways, you can gain similar advantages.

Not a good match for you? Without intermittent fasting, how to get in shape

When intermittent fasting isn't a good idea for you, how do you get in shape and lose weight?

Know the fundamentals of outstanding eating. It is by far the best thing for your health and wellness that you can do.

Cook and eat food in its entirety. Regularly workout. Remain consistent. And if you want some guidance doing all that, find a mentor or a coach.

Heck, even if you decide to pursue intermittent fasting, that last part is true.

Although self-experimentation is fine, even better is guided experimentation, especially when an experienced coach is supervising it.

CHAPTER 2

THE ADVANTAGES OF
INTERMITTENT FASTING

1. Weight Loss

Most individuals start to lose weight with IF. And at least in the short term, that claim appears to hold up. There is a chance that any version of IF may contribute to weight loss, according to an article published in August 2015 in the Journal of the Academy of Nutrition and Dietetics. The researchers examined data from 13 studies and found that for a two-week trial, the average weight loss ranged from 1.3% to 8% for an eight-week trial.

If you're hoping to quickly lose weight, that's probably welcome news, but the fact that those studies were short-term means it's unclear whether IF is sustainable and can help you keep extra pounds off in the long run.

The other catch: The amount of weight loss does not seem to be any more than what you would expect from another calorie-restricted diet, and you could even end up gaining weight depending on how many calories you eat per day. The diet does not restrict high-calorie foods, after all.

When the diet is done correctly, Dr Lowden says that IF can be as effective as normal caloric restriction. Some people, particularly busy people who have no time to devote to meal planning, may even find it easier to follow a time-restricted diet than something like the keto diet or the paleo diet, she says.

2. Reduced blood pressure

In the short term, IF may aid in lowering high blood pressure. Research published in Diet and Healthy Aging in June 2018 showed that 16:8 significantly lowered systolic blood pressure among the 23 participants in the study. According to a study published in March 2019 in Nutrients, the relation has been shown in both animal and human studies. And IF led to even greater reductions in systolic blood pressure than another diet that did not require fixed eating hours, a study published in the European Journal of Nutrition in October 2019 found.

It is crucial to have healthy blood pressure-unhealthy levels can increase the risk of heart disease, stroke, and kidney disease.

But the study so far shows that these blood pressure advantages last only when IF is being exercised. Researchers found that the blood pressure readings returned to their original levels after the diet ended, and individuals returned to eating normally.

3. Reduced Inflammation

Animal studies have shown that inflammation levels can be reduced by both IF and general calorie restriction, although clinical trials are few and far between. Fifty participants who were fasting for Ramadan, the Muslim holiday, which includes fasting from sunrise to sunset, and eating overnight, were involved in the study. The study showed that pro-inflammatory markers were lower than usual during the fasting period, blood pressure, body weight, and body fat.

4. Decreased cholesterol

Alternate-day fasting may help lower total

cholesterol and LDL cholesterol when done in combination with endurance exercise, according to a three-week-long study published in obesity. "According to the Centers for Disease Control and Prevention, LDL cholesterol is the "bad cholesterol that can increase the danger of heart disease or stroke. According to the Mayo Clinic, researchers also noted that IF decreases the presence of triglycerides, which are fats found in the blood that can result in stroke, heart attack, or heart disease. One caveat here the research was brief, so more research is needed to understand whether the cholesterol effects of IF are long-lasting.

5. Better Stroke Survivors Outcomes

To help reduce your risk of stroke, healthier cholesterol levels and lower blood pressure (two advantages noted above) play a major role. But that isn't the only possible advantage of IF related to stroke. An article in Experimental and Translational Stroke Medicine found that a protective mechanism for the brain may be provided by IF and calorie reduction in general. It seems that eating this pre-stroke may prevent brain injury in cases where the stroke occurs. The researchers say that future studies are needed to determine whether the recovery can be aided by following IF post-stroke.

6. Brain feature boosted

Dr Gottfried says that IF can boost attention and mental acuity. And there is some early evidence to support that idea: A study published in Experimental Biology and Medicine in February 2018 on rats showed that it could help protect against the loss in memory that comes with age. IF can strengthen ties in the brain's hippocampus and also protect against amyloid plaques seen in Alzheimer's patients, according to the Johns Hopkins Health Study. However, this research was conducted only on animals, so it is still uncertain if the advantage holds humans.

7. Cancer Protection

According to a review of research published in The American Journal of Clinical Nutrition, some studies have shown that alternate-day fasting can reduce cancer risk by decreasing lymphoma development, limiting tumour survival, and slowing the spread of cancer cells.

However, all animal studies were the studies that showed the cancer benefit, and further research is needed to confirm an advantage for humans and explain the mechanism behind these results.

8. Cell Turnover Increased

In other words, a break from eating and digestion allows the body a chance to regenerate and get rid of the garbage inside the cells that can accelerate ageing, she says. Gottfried says that the time of rest involved in intermittent fasting improves autophagy, which is a crucial detoxification function in the body to clean out damaged cells."

A study published in Nutrients in May 2019 found that time-restricted feeding increased the expression of the autophagy gene LC3A and the protein mTOR, which regulates cell growth, which the researchers described as eating between 8 a.m. and 2 p.m. This study was limited, involving four days for only 11 participants. Another research published in Autophagy in August 2019 also noted that food restriction is a well-recognized way to improve autophagy, specifically neuronal autophagy, which can provide the brain with protective benefits. However, there were still some limitations with this study: it was performed on mice and not humans.

9. Reduced Insulin Resistance

In people with diabetes, Gottfried suggests that intermittent fasting may help stabilize blood sugar levels because it resets insulin, although more research is needed. According to a study published in Nutrients in April 2019, the idea is that restricting calories might improve insulin resistance, which is a marker of type 2 diabetes. Fasting, such as the IF-associated type of fasting, encourages a drop in insulin levels, which will play a role in reducing the risk for type 2, the study notes. In other facilities, I have colleagues who have seen positive results, particularly in improving insulin needs for diabetics," Lowden says."

This effect was investigated in humans in the study above published in Nutrition and Healthy Aging. While a 16:8 approach resulted in reductions in insulin resistance, the results were not significantly different from those of the control group. And this study again was small.

Registered dietitians advise individuals with diabetes to cautiously approach intermittent fasting. There may be a higher risk of low blood sugar, which can be life-threatening, for people on certain type 2 diabetes medications or those on insulin (whether to manage blood sugar for type 2 or type 1 diabetes). Check with your doctor if you have any type of diabetes before trying intermittent fasting, they advise.

10. Higher risk of cardiovascular issues

According to the Nutrients report, as insulin levels decrease, the risk of serious cardiovascular events, such as congestive heart failure, is also significant for patients with type 2 diabetes since, according to the American Heart Association, they are two to four times more likely than adults without diabetes to die from heart disease.

Although there are no human studies to validate the effect, observational studies have shown that IF can provide both cardiovascular and metabolic benefits, the Nutrients study noted. Low suspects that metabolic parameter changes, such as lower triglyceride levels and a decrease in blood sugar levels, resulting from weight loss and would be achieved regardless of how the weight was lost, for example, whether through IF or a low-carb diet.

11. Increased longevity

A few animal and rodent studies have shown that IF can extend the life span, possibly because fasting appears to build resistance to age-related diseases. In June 2019, a review published in Current Obesity Reports noted that while these findings are promising, they have been difficult to replicate in human studies. It's better to be sceptical about this potential advantage until that happens.

12.   A Better Night Sleep

You know that diet can affect wakefulness and sleepiness if you've ever felt like you fell into a food coma after a large meal. As a result of practising this way of eating, some IF supporters report being able to sleep better. "Sleep may be affected by IF and mealtimes," Rose-Francis says. About why?

One theory is that IF influences the circadian rhythm, which defines the rhythms of sleep. A controlled circadian rhythm means that you can easily fall asleep and wake up feeling refreshed, but according to an article published in Nature and Science of Sleep in December 2018, research to support this theory is limited.

The other hypothesis focuses that by the time you hit the pillow, getting your last meal earlier in the evening means you would have digested the food. According to the National Sleep Foundation, digestion is better accomplished while you're standing, and going to sleep with a full stomach can lead to acid reflux or heartburn at bedtime, which can make it difficult to fall asleep.

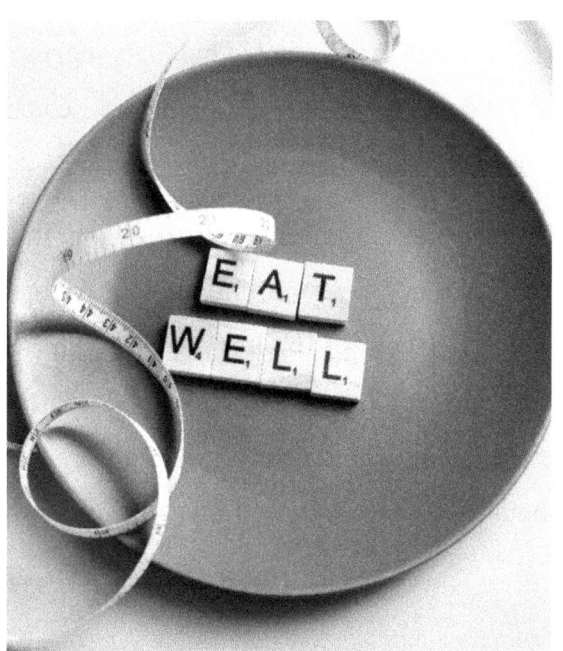

CHAPTER 3

THE SCIENCE BEHIND FASTING INTERMITTENTLY AND HOW TO MAKE IT WORK FOR YOU

W hile there is scientific evidence for intermittent fasting advantages, according to leading researcher Satchin Panda, it is neither a quick nor a guaranteed fix. Panda, a professor of circadian biology at La Jolla, California's Salk Institute for Biological Studies, spent his career studying the human body's complex biochemical processes. His research in mice and individuals suggests that intermittent fasting, including weight loss, could benefit human health in various ways.

Let's put one thing up front before diving into science: there isn't one way to do intermittent fasting. You will find a menu of options, each with its proponents, if you google it. There is the 5: 2 diet for two days of the week, which involves eating very few calories (about 500-600) followed by five days of normal eating. Or there is alternate-day fasting, which means eating normally and then the next eating either nothing or just 500 calories.

In essence, all intermittent fasting methods are based on the same idea: Your body will use its stored fat for energy when you reduce your caloric intake. But the possibility that it is easier for people to limit calories for limited periods rather than for the days, weeks, and months required by conventional diets makes intermittent fasting different from simply cutting calories. Plus, there may be additional positive effects of the particular type of intermittent fasting that Panda has studied.

Panda has focused on the technique of intermittent fasting, known as time-limited eating. In this format, within an 8-to-12-hour window, a person consumes all of their calories for the day. Let's say that you usually start your day at 7 a.m. with the first cup of coffee and eventually wind down around 11 p.m. with popcorn and a drink. You could switch to eating breakfast at am, including coffee, time-restricted eating, and finishing your dinner by 6 p.m. That way, within 10 hours, you consume all your meals, and you most definitely forgo calories from desserts, evening snacks, and alcohol. But that's not the story as a whole.

It seems that time-restricted feeding does more for the body than merely reducing the consumption of calories. A 2012 research that Panda and colleagues did with mice first suggested this. They took two genetically identical sets of mice and fed them the same diet, which is low in protein, high in fat and simple sugar and a lab-mice version of the standard American diet.

Although both groups were given the same amount of food, one group had access to food for 24 hours, and then the other group had access to food for only 8 hours. Mice are nocturnal, usually sleeping during the day and feeding at night. But when one group was given access to food round-the-clock, those mice started eating some of it during the day as well, when they would normally sleep.

The mice who were able to eat at all hours showed signs of insulin resistance after 18 weeks and had liver damage. But there were no such conditions for the mice who ate in the 8-hour window. They also weighed 28%

less than mice with 24-hour food access, even though both groups consumed the same number of calories a day. "It was an earth-shattering kind of thing," Panda recalls. Until then, he said that he and other researchers had thought that the total number of calories was what determined weight gain, rather than when they were eaten.

With three extra sets of mice, his team repeated the experiment and got the same results. For different food types and for eating windows of up to 15 hours, the results were also steady, although, interestingly, the shorter the window, the less weight the mice gained. They also gained less weight when the time-restricted mice were switched to unrestricted feeding for two days a week or what Panda calls "having the weekend off," than the mice allowed to eat 24 hours a day.

Panda's team then tried another way: they took mice that had gained weight due to unrestricted feeding and switched them to time-restricted eating. Those mice lost weight and maintained it for 12 weeks until the end of the study, despite eating the same calories. They also decreased their insulin resistance, which is believed to be related to obesity, although the association is still not understood by scientists. Of course, the human body is more complicated than a mouse, says Panda, but these experiments were the first indication of how vital timing could be when it comes to how our bodies use food.

Scientists have discovered in recent years that so many of the functions of the human body are related to our circadian rhythms. For instance, most of us know that getting sunlight early in the morning is beneficial to our sleep and mood and that exposure to light from our mobile phones or laptops at 9 p.m. will interrupt the sleep of our night. "Similarly, food can nurture us at the right time, and healthy food can be junk food at the wrong time," Panda says. It is processed as fat instead of fuel, which makes sense if you explore the fundamentals of how human metabolism operates.

Time-restricted intake provides our body with more time to use up fat. Our body uses carbohydrates for energy when we feed, and if we do not need them right away, they are stored as glycogen in the liver or turned into fat. Our body tends to function on glucose from the carbohydrates that we've just consumed for a few hours before tapping into stored glycogen, or carbohydrates, in the liver after we've completed eating for the day. The glycogen lasts for several hours, which is when our body starts to tap into its stored fat, before running out about eight hours after we stop feeding.

In this fat-burning mode of our metabolism, we spend longer as we shorten our eating window and prolong our fasting window. But we turn back to the other mode and start burning carbohydrates and storing glycogen and fat when we eat food again, even if it's just coffee with a bit of sugar and milk. So if you finish eating your evening snack at 10 p.m., your body will run out of glycogen at around 6 a.m. and start burning fat. You have given your body three extra hours to use fat as fuel if you normally eat breakfast at 6 a.m., but you change it to 9 a.m.

Panda followed up on his time-limited human eating tests and found there was potential there too. He and his peers attempted to place small groups of people for 16 weeks on a time-restricted eating plan in 2015. Interestingly, the researchers offered no diet instructions or guidance to these individuals at all.

Instead, the subjects were told to select a window of 10-to-12 hours to do all their feeding. They took photos of their food as they ate and texted it to the researchers. The subjects displayed a small amount of weight loss after 16 weeks-an an average of just over 8 pounds each. But according to Panda, they reported having a better sleep, more energy in the mornings, and less hunger at bedtime, implying that time-restricted eating "actually has a systemic impact throughout the body." While a sample of individuals was far too small to draw conclusive conclusions, the researchers found it reassuring that this basic intervention appeared easy to introduce and maintain for subjects.

Some potential for avoiding diabetes has been demonstrated by time-restricted feeding. In a study of 15 men at risk for type 2 diabetes conducted by Panda, he and his team found that the men displayed a lower blood glucose spike after a test meal, a sign of increased insulin sensitivity, after one week of limiting them to eating within a nine-hour window. It could help lower cholesterol as well. Panda and colleagues had 19 individuals in another trial, most of whom were on medication to reduce cholesterol or blood pressure or treat diabetes, limiting their eating time. They lowered their overall cholesterol by an average of around 11% after 12 weeks of eating within a 10-hour window.

What's more, Panda checked in one year later and found that in an 8-11 hour span, approximately 3⁄4 of the subjects were still voluntarily eating. "It was gratifying that for some time, they were able to self-sustain this," Panda says. This is good news, given that 1⁄3 to 1⁄2 of dieters ultimately regain more weight than they lose, by some figures.

According to Panda, here is how you can practice time-restricted feeding. Although some intermittent fasting plans allow people to have unlimited amounts of coffee and tea during the day, he says you should eat only water during your fasting window. This means no tea, coffee, or herbal tea, all of which can alter the blood's chemistry, which is why medical blood tests are not permitted during fasts.

After you wake up, Panda suggests you drink plain hot water; it can give you some of the same calming feelings as coffee. Of course, he says it's OK to have some black coffee if you must be alert in the morning but stay away from any added sugar, honey, creamer, or other sweeteners. "Just a teaspoon of sugar is enough to double our blood sugar," he says, which transforms the body back into carb-burning mode out of fat-burning mode.

When to have your meals, Panda suggests that you wait until you've been up for a few hours to eat breakfast. The hormone cortisol spikes and high cortisol levels can impede your glucose regulation about 45 minutes after you wake up. Plus, just about two hours after waking, the hormone melatonin, which prepares our body for sleep, wears off. This implies that your pancreas, which generates the insulin required to use carbohydrates in the food, is just only waking up for those first two hours. Then around two to three hours before bedtime, you should try to finish your last meal because that's when melatonin starts to prepare your body, including your pancreas, for sleep.

While intermittent fasting, and in particular time-restricted feeding, holds tantalizing promise, it's still early days. Other study groups have backed up some of his findings since Panda started his research. Research published in Cell Metabolism in July, for example, showed that individuals on a time-restricted eating program lowered their calorie consumption, even though they were not asked to, and lost a small amount of weight.

There's a need for more time-restricted eating studies. So far, no research has been conducted on human subjects that have lasted longer than a few months. Researchers often need to know how the human body is affected by fasting. For example, in mice that limit their eating to an eight-nine hour window, the gut microbiome has been shown to adjust such that they digest nutrients differently, consuming less sugar and fat. In humans, is this possible? To be seen, that remains. Panda is not the only one who explores the benefits of time-restricted eating that go beyond weight loss; other researchers are now starting to examine whether intermittent fasting can protect the brain from neurodegenerative diseases as well.

For weight loss, intermittent fasting is not a magic bullet. Some research also indicates that individuals who follow the 5:2 diet or alternate-day fasting can instinctively eat more or decrease their behaviour on fasting days before and after their fasting days, negating the benefits of calorie reduction. In his time-restricted eating experiments, Panda says that after taking the concept of eating whatever they wanted within a window to the limit, he saw some participants gain weight, bingeing on the foods they normally abstained from. The human body may also have ways of slowing down metabolism, unlike rodents, such that you also burn less when you eat fewer calories. Finally, it is uncertain if intermittent fasting is effective for individuals who do not lose weight. In reality, for individuals who struggle with binge-eating disorder or anorexia, there is a possible danger; it is not difficult to see how attempting intermittent fasting could promote these dangerous behaviours.

There are practical benefits to time-restricted eating over other dieting options: It is simple and available. Many individuals do not have the time or money to count calories, schedule their meals, purchase those foods, and count their calories. Hence, diets are mostly the luxury of individuals who can afford them. Anyone who can count time and limit drinking and eating to particular hours can do time-restricted eating.

Panda and his colleagues are now carrying out an analysis of time-restricted eating for 120 participants. They're also investigating if, by eating in a 10-hour window, firefighters could improve their health. Because of their circadian cycles' frequent disturbance, firefighters and other shift workers are more vulnerable to disease. (Note from the editor: If you want to participate in the research of Panda, download a free app that will ask you to record your sleep, exercise, drugs, and anything you eat and drink. Seven groups of scientists worldwide are also currently doing research using the framework of the app.)

People who want to lose weight have had to concentrate on changing their everyday menus for a long time. Time-restricted eating can increase the variables that we can regulate. "We have a menu of options when it comes to health," says Panda, who adheres to a 10-hour feeding window. "We can now add the meal schedule to the menu."

CHAPTER 4
UNDERSTANDING AUTOPHAGY

Autophagy means self-eating, but this is a positive thing, rest assured. Autophagy is how your body cleanses damaged cells and toxins and helps you regenerate new healthier cells.

Our cells accumulate a range of dead organelles, damaged proteins, and oxidized particles over time that obstruct the body's inner workings. This speeds up the symptoms of ageing and age-related diseases because cells do not naturally divide and function.

Because many of our cells need to last a lifetime, like those in the brain, the body has developed a unique way to rid itself of those faulty parts and naturally defend itself against disease.

HOW AUTOPHAGY WORKS

Think of your body as a kitchen. You clean up the counter after making a meal, throw away the leftovers, and recycle some of the food. You've got a tidy kitchen the next day. In your body, this is autophagy doing its thing and doing it well.

Think about the same scenario now, except you are older and not as powerful. You leave the leftovers on the counter after preparing your dinner. Some of it goes down in the landfill, some of it doesn't. On the counter, the waste, and the recycling bin, the scraps remain. They never open the door to the dumpster, and in your kitchen, radioactive waste begins to build up. There is food fermentation on the floor, and all sorts of unpleasant smells wafting out the door.

You have a tough time keeping up with the daily grime due to the onslaught of pollutants and toxins. This situation is close to autophagy, which doesn't work as well as it should.

In maintenance mode, autophagy normally hums along quietly behind the scenes. It plays a part in how the body reacts to stress periods, maintains equilibrium, and controls cell function.

There is proof that you slow down the ageing process, reduce inflammation, and improve your overall performance when you cause autophagy. You will naturally increase your autophagy response to help your body resist disease and encourage longevity (more on that later).

LONGEVITY AND AUTOPHAGY

Because of our ability to adapt to biological stressors, humans have evolved to live longer, from physical exercise to starvation. Research from the Newcastle University study[4] found that this ability is due to minor changes in an autophagy-inducing protein known as p62.

Protein p62 activates to induce autophagy or begin cleaning by sensing the metabolic byproducts that trigger cell damage (called reactive oxygen species ROS). In particular, all the damaged products that have accumulated in your body are eliminated by p62 proteins so that you are better able to manage biological stress. A direct consequence of the p62 protein doing its thing during autophagy is homeostasis (balanced cellular function) and vibrant health. As a consequence, fresh cell development is handed over to the weakened products that build up in your body over time, and this is what keeps you safe.

While humans have this ability, lower species, such as fruit flies, do not. Therefore, the research team set out to find the part of human protein p62 that enables ROS to be sensed. With "humanized" p62, they then developed genetically modified fruit flies. Outcome? The "humanized" flies have survived in adverse environments for longer.

"This tells us that skills may have evolved to allow better stress resistance and a longer lifespan, such as sensing stress and activating protective processes such as autophagy," says Dr Viktor Korolchuk, lead author of the report.

WHAT ARE THE ADVANTAGES OF AUTOPHAGY?

The main advantages of autophagy seem to come in the form of the principles of anti-ageing. In reality, Petre says that turning the clock back and producing younger cells is best known as the body's way.

Khorana points out that to protect us, autophagy is enhanced when our cells are stressed, improving the lifespan.

Also, registered dietitian Scott Keatley, RD, CDN, says that autophagy keeps the body working in times of hunger by breaking down cellular material and reusing it for required processes.

"This requires energy, of course, and can not continue forever, but it gives us more time to find food," he adds.

Petre says at the cellular level that the advantages of autophagy include:

- Toxic proteins linked to neurodegenerative disorders such as Parkinson's and Alzheimer's disease are eliminated from cells.

- Residual protein recycling

- Providing cells with energy and building blocks that could still benefit from repair

- It encourages regeneration and healthy cells on a bigger scale.

Autophagy is gaining a lot of attention for the role it can play in cancer prevention or care, too.

When we age, autophagy decreases because this

means that cells that no longer function or can harm can multiply, which is the MO of cancer cells," Keatley explains."

While all cancers start with some kind of defective cells, Petre says the body, often using autophagic processes, should recognize and remove those cells. That's why some researchers are looking at the possibility that cancer risk could be lowered by autophagy.

Although there is no scientific evidence to confirm this, Petre says some studies indicate that many cancer cells can be removed by autophagy.

"She explains, "This is how the body polices cancer villains. "The recognition and destruction of what went wrong and the triggering of the repair mechanism helps to reduce the risk of cancer."

Researchers conclude that new research will contribute to knowledge that will assist them in targeting autophagy as a cancer treatment.

Diet modifications that can improve autophagy

Note that autophagy simply means "self-eating."

Therefore it makes sense that it is understood that intermittent fasting and ketogenic diets induce autophagy.

Fasting is the most efficient way to cause autophagy Petre explains."

"Ketosis, a high fat and low carbohydrate diet provide the same benefits of fasting without fasting, such as a shortcut that induces the same beneficial metabolic changes," she says. "It gives the body a break by not overwhelming the body with an external load to focus on its health and repair."

You get about 75% of your daily calories from fat in the keto diet and 5 to 10 % of your calories from carbs.

This change in calorie sources causes the metabolic pathways of your body to change. Instead of the glucose that is extracted from carbohydrates, it will start using fat for food.

Your body will start making ketone bodies that have several protective effects in response to this restriction. Khorana says studies indicate that Ketosis, which has neuroprotective functions, can also cause starvation-induced autophagy.

'In both diets, low glucose levels occur and are related to low insulin and high levels of glucagon,' explains Petre. And the level of glucagon is the one that initiates autophagy.

"Through fasting or ketosis, when the body is low on sugar, it brings positive stress that wakes up the survival repair mode," she adds.

Exercise is one non-diet area that may also play a role in inducing autophagy. According to one animal study, physical exercise can cause autophagy in organs that are part of metabolic control procedures.

The muscles, liver, pancreas, and adipose tissue may be included in this.

Fasting Connect

Autophagy happens naturally inside the body, but many people wonder whether they can use particular stimuli to cause autophagy.

Fasting is a potential autophagic cause. For long periods, hours, or even a day or more, they willingly go without food when someone fasts.

Fasting varies from conventional limits on calories. They decrease their daily intake of food when a person reduces their calories. Depending on how much food a person eats during feeding times, fasting can or may not result in calorie restriction.

A 2018 review of the current study strongly indicates that autophagy can be caused by both fasting and calorie restriction.

While there is some evidence of this process happening in humans, non-human animals were involved in most of these studies.

The cells of the body are put under stress by fasting and calorie restriction. If a person reduces the amount of food that goes into their body, they get fewer calories from their cells, than they need to function properly.

The cells must function more effectively when this occurs. Autophagy allows the body cells to clean out and recycle any unwanted or damaged parts in response to the stress brought about by fasting or calorie restriction.

Scientists are unsure about which cells, however,

react in this way to fasting and calorie restriction. People who want to induce autophagy by fasting should be conscious that, for instance, this does not target fat cells.

Researchers are still debating whether fasting in the brain will cause autophagy. At least one animal study shows that autophagy in brain cells may be caused by short-term fasting.

How can you cause autophagy?

By placing cells under tension, fasting, and calorie restriction both cause autophagy. Researchers suspect, however, that other ways to induce autophagy can exist.

Exercise

Exercise also brings the cells of the body under tension. The components of their cells become weakened and inflamed when individuals exercise. The authors of one paper explain that with autophagy, our cells react to this problem.

This indicates that to cause autophagy, people might be able to use the exercise. Indeed there is evidence that exercise in human skeletal muscles improves autophagy.

Curcumin

Scientists have also proposed that, at least in experiments involving mice, curcumin consumption causes autophagy. Curcumin is a naturally occurring chemical found in the root of turmeric, a globally common spice.

One animal research, for example, indicated that curcumin-induced autophagy restoration could protect against diabetic cardiomyopathy, a heart muscle condition that affects individuals with diabetes.

Another research in mice showed that curcumin helped combat cognitive dysfunction by inducing autophagy in some brain regions due to chemotherapy.

While these preliminary results are encouraging, it is important to remember that further research is needed before scientists can draw any conclusions. Scientists do not yet know, in particular, whether increasing intake of curcumin can cause autophagy in humans.

HERE ARE THE 3 MAIN WAYS TO IMPROVE THE BODY'S AUTOPHAGY.

1. Reduce your carb intake

Without forgoing your favourite rib eye, there's a great way to activate autophagy, although you'll probably need to quit candy.

Ketosis is named. The concept is to reduce carbohydrates to such low levels that there is no choice for the body but to use fat as a source of fuel. This is the magic behind the ketogenic diet that is wildly popular.

Keto foods are low in carbohydrates and high in fat (steak, bacon, and peanut butter shakes are a bonus for the keto crowd). Of your total calories, between 60 and 70 % come from fat.

Protein accounts for 20 to 30 % of calories, while carbs are responsible for just 5 %.

Being in Ketosis while maintaining muscle can help people lose body fat. There is some evidence that it can also help the body fight cancerous tumours, reduce the risk of diabetes, and protect it from brain disorders and epilepsy. Trustworthy Source

Indeed, rats fed a keto diet in a 2018 study had less brain damage during seizures.

"Champ says, Ketosis is like an autophagic hack. "Without actually fasting, you get a lot of the same metabolic modifications and benefits of fasting."

If it sounds too hard to remain in Ketosis, then take heart. Similar advantages in people who adopted a diet in which no more than 30% of their total calories came from carbs were noted in a 2012 report, Champ says.

Note: Before starting a keto diet, anyone with health problems, especially kidney or liver problems, should talk with a doctor.

2. Try intermittent fasting

Another stressful act that the body does not love immediately but eventually profits from is missing meals. Research has shown that tons of good stuff occasionally happen quickly.

One research review showed that intermittent fasting and autophagy could make cancer more successful while maintaining normal cells and reducing side effects.

Intermittent fasting has been shown in another mouse study to promote cognitive performance, brain structure, and neuroplasticity, which is fancy-speak for the brain's capacity to reorganize and repair itself.

That said, if autophagy was the cause, it wasn't totally clear. Plus, on mice, the analysis was completed. You may have learned about a certain Twitter account with an issue with people who speak a lot about mouse science.

Give fasting a shot in the meantime. Although Champ fasts a few days a week for 18 hours a day, he knows it can be a difficult regimen for most of us.

Various variations of intermittent fasting appear to show pretty awesome health benefits. An analysis of the study concluded that it could have several beneficial effects, ranging from a healthy weight of the body and a reduced risk of cancer to an extended lifespan. Trustworthy Source

Bear in mind that for children, for certain people with diabetes or other blood sugar problems, or pregnant women, fasting is usually not recommended.

3. Regularly exercise

If you have not been tipped off by sweating, grunting, and post-workout pain, here's the deal: exercise puts stress on your body.

Working out hurts your muscles, producing microscopic tears that your body then rushes to repair. It makes the muscles stronger and more immune to any more "damage" you might cause them.

Daily exercise is the most common way for individuals to accidentally help cleanse their bodies. (So that fresh, refreshed feeling you get after working out has substance to it.)

In 2012 looked at autophagosomes, structures that form around pieces of cells that the body has chosen to recycle. Scientists noticed something fascinating after engineering mice to have glowing green autophagosomes (as one does).

After they exercised for 30 minutes on a treadmill, the mice's pace was healthily demolishing their cells dramatically increased. Until the little guys had run for 80 minutes, the rate continued to grow.

What about humans, then?

The amount of exercise needed to turn on the autophagic boost is difficult to find out.

[These are currently difficult questions to address," says Daniel Klionsky, PhD, a cell biologist who specializes in autophagy at the University of Michigan." "Exercise has many advantages, aside from the possible role of autophagy."

Is there an easier way?

Still not. But if researchers can distil the advantages of autophagy into a pill, there's a lot of money to be made, so you can be sure they're trying.

"Of course, because it would be easier than dieting, people are looking for ways to induce autophagy through chemicals," Klionsky says but warns that we're a long way off.

Champ observes that anti-epileptic medications already exist that imitate Ketosis.

For example, Stiripentol was approved by the FDA in 2018 and can mimic the effects of a ketogenic diet. It is used to treat seizures associated with a rare type of epilepsy, Dravet syndrome.

Don't get your hopes up yet. "There are plenty metabolic changes that take place during ketosis that it might not be possible to mimic all of them with a pill," Champ says. "For the benefits, the body stress that comes with entering ketosis could be necessary."

Just remember: to enjoy these benefits, you don't have to remain in Ketosis, fast, or exercise vigorously all day, every day. Just a few hours can be useful here and there.

Female hormones can be disrupted by intermittent fasting.

Experimenting with intermittent fasting probably seems tiny in the grand scheme of health decisions. So what was it going to hurt to give it a shot?

Well, it's a bigger deal for some women than you might expect. It turns out that the hormones controlling key functions are extraordinarily responsive to your energy intakes, such as ovulation, metabolism, and even mood. In reality, changing how much you eat can adversely affect your reproductive hormones.

CHAPTER 5
INTERMITTENTLY FASTING AND REPRODUCTIVE HORMONES

O ne way that fasting affects reproductive hormones has to do with something called the hypothalamic-pituitary-gonadal axis in both women and men. This is, thankfully, more commonly referred to as the HPG axis. In daily spurts, the hypothalamus releases the gonadotropin-releasing hormone (GnRH), called "pulses."

In daily spurts, the hypothalamus releases the gonadotropin-releasing hormone (GnRH), called "pulses."

2. GnRH pulses instruct the pituitary gland to release follicular stimulating hormone (LH) and luteinizing hormone (LH) (FSH).

3. Then, LH and FSH function on the gonads. In women, estrogen and progesterone production that we need to release a mature egg (ovulation) and to support pregnancy is stimulated by LH and FSH.

In males, they stimulate testosterone and sperm production. Because this chain of reactions occurs in women on a very specific, regular cycle, GnRH pulses need to be accurately timed, or everything can get out of whack. Eggs have not been published, cycles have ended... Here's the big takeaway: GnRH pulses seem to be very sensitive to environmental influences, and fasting can throw them off.

In some women, also short-term fasting, say, three days may change these hormonal pulses. There is also some evidence that skipping a single meal will start to put our hormonal system on alert, which of course, is not an emergency by itself. This may be why some women run into intermittent fasting issues. But why does eating less put alertness in our bodies? For many years scientists assumed that a woman's percentage of body fat regulated her reproductive system.

The idea was this: if your fat stores dipped below a certain amount, hormones would get mixed up, and your cycle would end somewhere about 11%.

Boom: no possibility of conception.

This has made a lot of sense from an evolutionary perspective. Our ancestors, who did not have access to Costco and Amazon, would be of major concern to have a low food supply. (Read: It wouldn't be a good time to give birth or raise young people.)

So if you were to lose body fat, your body might think that there's not much to eat and try to escape reproduction.

But the matter is more complex than that. Even before body fat drops, female bodies tend to go on alert.

Consequently, women who are not particularly lean can stop ovulating and lose their periods, too. That is why scientists now suspect that the overall energy balance may be more important for this process than the percentage of body fat, how many calories you eat versus how many you "burn."

How your diet can work against you, and too much stress.

You are known to be in a negative energy balance when you consistently consume less energy than you expend. How you lose weight is how you get into a negative energy balance. So this is exactly what many people are trying to accomplish by dieting. But in the context of other stressors, when it's extreme or goes on too long, it may be to blame for the hormonal spiral we see in some women who are fasting. Not only does negative energy equilibrium result from eating less food.

Also, it can result from:

- Poor nutrition

- An excessive amount of exercise

- Too much stress

- Infection, disease, chronic inflammation

- Too little rest and recovery

- Heck, by attempting to keep warm, we can even use up energy.

It may be enough for any combination of stressors to bring you into an unnecessary negative energy balance and avoid ovulation. For instance:

- too many days at the gym and not eating enough vegetables and fruits

- nursing flu and training for a marathon

- intermittent fasting and busting your butt to pay the mortgage

- You may be thinking, 'Did she just reference paying the mortgage?'

In harming your hormonal health, psychological stress may play a part.

Our bodies can't say the difference between our thoughts and feelings created by a real threat and something theoretical. (Such as thinking about how to get your abs.)

These "threats may increase our levels of the stress hormone cortisol." And with cortisol? It inhibits GnRH, our old friend.

Fast reminder: GnRH disruption causes a cascade effect that can inhibit the development of estrogen and progesterone hormones essential for reproduction in your ovaries.

So you might be hovering at 30% fat. But if you're in a negative energy balance for a long enough period, especially if you're very stressed, reproduction stops.

Why does intermittent fasting impact the hormones of women more than those of men?

We aren't completely sure.

When your dad/ brother/partner has been walking around looking ripped after doing intermittent fasting for a few months, we know: that's annoying to learn.

But there are several possible explanations for contributing:

1. Women may be more sensitive than men to changes in nutrient equilibrium.

When fasting or significantly restricting calories, men and women seem to respond differently. This may be due to kisspeptin, a molecule similar to a protein vital in the reproductive process.

Kisspeptin stimulates the production of GnRH in both sexes, and we understand that it is very susceptible to leptin, insulin, and ghrelin-hormones that control and respond to feelings of hunger and fullness.

Females have more kisspeptin than males,

interestingly. More kisspeptin may indicate that women's bodies are more susceptible to energy balance changes.

Fasting more readily causes women's production of kisspeptin to dip compared to men. It tosses GnRH off kilter12 when kisspeptin drops, which upsets the entire monthly hormonal cycle.

2. Compared with men, restricting certain nutrients such as protein may also have different effects on women.

Women tend to eat less protein than men in general And women who eat quickly usually eat even less protein (because they eat less overall).

That's an issue because protein provides amino acids that are critical for the process of reproduction.

If amino acids get too low, both your estrogen receptors and a hormone called insulin-like growth factor (IGF-1) can be negatively affected. During the menstrual cycle, both are needed to thicken the lining of the uterus. If the uterus's lining does not thicken, it is impossible to implant an egg, and pregnancy cannot occur.

Hence, low protein-diets can reduce fertility.

Why estrogen matters so much for a woman's appetite, mood, metabolism, and body fat.

Estrogen isn't just for reproduction and the uterus.

Throughout our bodies, we have estrogen receptors, including in our hearts, GI tract and bones.

Adjust the estrogen balance. Throughout this debate, you adjust metabolic functions: cognition, mood, digestion, regeneration, protein turnover, bone formation, appetite, and energy balance may be most important. Estrogens alter the peptides in the brain stem that tell you to feel full (cholecystokinin) or hungry (ghrelin).

Oestrogens also stimulate neurons in the hypothalamus that halt the production of peptides that regulate appetite.

Do something that causes your estrogen to reduce (like fast), and you might feel a lot hungrier than you would under normal circumstances, and eat a lot more.

Oestrogen affects the storage of fat, too.

Oestrogens are vital metabolic regulators, as you can see.

Yes, plural, estrogenic. Three different estrogen types found in the body are estriol, estradiol, and estrone, also known as estrogenic metabolites.

Over time, the proportions of these Oestrogens change. Estradiol is the major player before menopause. But estradiol drops after menopause, whereas estrone stays about the same. It remains unclear the exact roles of each of these estrogens. But some theorize that a decrease in estradiol may cause an increase in the storage of fat. This could at least explain why some women find it harder to lose fat after menopause.

The theory does not, however, explain anything. Although a decrease in estradiol may be associated with an increase in fat storage, it is probably not the only cause (and might not be causal at all).

Instead, fat increases around menopause may be due to ageing, reduced muscle mass, and appetite changes; more generally, low estradiol is also associated with higher appetite).

So intermittent fasting in women for weight loss... is complicated.

Because... Women's bodies could just be more susceptible to energy balance shifts.

And And...

It can disturb the HPG axis when our bodies sense shifts, and our whole hormonal cycle is thrown away. If other stressors are wasting our resources, this hormonal turmoil can be exacerbated further.

(Think the family hamster might be "lost" in the heating ducts... maybe all at the same time, taking care of children, working more to get the promotion, coping with a chronic injury.) Intermittent fasting can minimize estrogen, and reduced estrogen can improve the storage of appetite and fat. So, fasting to control your weight? Maybe it's kinda... counterproductive. The more you struggle, the harder it gets, like being caught in one of those Chinese finger traps.

Intermittent Fasting Through The Lifetime Of Females

Women, childbearing or not, go through many different stages of existence, marked by major hormonal alteration.

Such hormonal changes can have major physical and psychological impacts and affect sleep, digestion, reactivity to stress, and metabolism.

Here are a couple of those stages and how they may be affected by intermittent fasting.

Intermittent fasting in girls and teens

Fasting is not recommended during times of intense development, including childhood and adolescence. Many kids are born with the ability to monitor their food consumption reasonably well, provided they are given a variety of healthy choices to choose from.

Teenagehood (and even earlier) may be a time of extreme self-scrutiny and social comparison and is often considered "dieting" by many young girls. It is a sensitive time, even when it is necessary to change eating habits. Focus on growing appetite awareness and conscious eating, and prioritizing whole, nutritious foods instead of restricting food. Promoting an enjoyable, stress-free relationship with food and a kind, compassionate relationship with the body as much as possible.

Intermittent Ovulation And Fasting

Intermittent fasting might make things complicated if you're trying to conceive.

Ovulation can be inhibited by fasting. No egg is released if you're not ovulating. It can't be fertilized if no egg gets released.

Doctors or other health practitioners may have advised certain women to lose weight before becoming pregnant. Many women are starting to think more critically about their health while contemplating pregnancy and view weight loss as a step in this direction.

Whatever the justification for considering intermittent fasting, remember this For hormonal equilibrium, intermittent fasting is not the right protocol for weight loss to suggest for most women.

Most women do well with moderate, sustainable, good eating behaviours in the reproductive phase of life.

Unless a woman is paid to look or act in a certain way (such as a physical competitor or a professional athlete), it may not be worth sacrificing fertility and hormonal balance.

When Pregnant, Intermittent Fasting

Pregnancy is like childhood and adolescence, a period of intense development.

Weight gain is a desirable consequence of developing pregnancy and is a symbol of a stable, growing infant.

Even though weight gain is needed during this period, the upward-creeping scale makes many women uncomfortable. During this time, women who are extremely body-conscious or want to lose weight before pregnancy can also think about weight loss.

Some women may also be recommended to control their weight during pregnancy by a doctor. (Which is a lot to ask when you feel nauseous and exhausted and anxious about changing, you know, your entire life.)

Even if a medical professional proposes weight loss, fasting during this period is not suitable.

Focus on increasing nutrition instead of limiting food: striving to get sufficient protein, healthy fats, quality carbohydrates, colourful vegetables, and fruits. (And if you can just eat bread and pickles from your topsy-turvy stomach, that's great. Do your best and take a prenatal multivitamin.)

You can also boost health and control weight gain by exercising, given that your doctor has cleared you. We have an infographic for that too if you're curious about what to do: how to exercise during pregnancy.

When Breastfeeding, Intermittent Fasting

If you have a baby and decide to breastfeed, you already know that this is a challenging time for your body: you might still be recovering from childbirth, you're probably deprived of sleep, and you've flipped around all your life. Plus, the baby is now treating you like a buffet of all-you-can-drinks.

Your body requires extra nurturing, extra nutrients, and less stress during this time. For these reasons, for breastfeeding women, intermittent fasting is probably not a good protocol.

Many moms worry about "losing the weight of the baby" and may feel pressured and impatient to get back their "pre-baby" body. Women can lose weight during this time, but more moderate approaches are safer and will probably yield better long-term results.

Try a moderate exercise (stroller walking counts!) and portion management for safe, sustainable weight loss.

In Ageing Females, Intermittent Fasting

Puberty, menstruation, perhaps pregnancy, and postpartum. Just what a rollercoaster.

Then comes menopause, another hormonal transition point that can stir us up physically, psychologically, and socially in women's lives.

After decades of being dedicated to children, spouses, and careers, women may return to themselves in this phase. Or they may be busier than ever before, looking after ageing parents and young adult children. (The one who's just. Won't. Move. Out.)

Increasing age often triggers a desire to concentrate on health, whatever the context.

Because of its association with longevity, some women are interested in intermittent fasting. In an uncomplicated way, others just want to lose fat.

While we do not have quality science on whether intermittent fasting is beneficial to menopausal or postmenopausal women, we know that it is also a stressor to restrict food.

Women who are concerned with controlling body weight control food intake tend to have higher levels of cortisol than women who do not. Connect that to the sleep disturbances that are so normal in menopause, and your "stress bucket" gets pretty full.

Lower levels of estrogen also mean that your body has a reduced ability to cope with stress. That bucket is filling up faster than it used to be.

Although many stressors, such as exercise, learning, and change, are good for us, they only make us stronger if we permit ourselves to recover from them.

So, if you're a woman in this phase, try intermittent

fasting only if:

- You're getting quality sleep.

- Your stress is low.

- You don't have any nutrient deficiencies.

- You are not tormented by hot flashes and mood swings.

So for women, is intermittent fasting bad?

All right, not necessarily.

Surely, however, fasting is not for everyone. And the truth is some women are not even supposed to bother experimenting. Do not attempt intermittent fasting if:

- You are pregnant •

- You have a history of eating disorders.

- You're under chronic stress

- You're not sleeping well.

- You're new to exercise and diet.

Pregnant women have additional energy requirements. So if you start a family, it's not a good idea for intermittent fasting.

Ditto if you have chronic stress or if you don't sleep well. Your body requires nurturing, not extra stress.

And if you've suffered in the past (or are currently dealing with disordered eating), you probably understand that a fasting regimen could lead you down a path that could cause more problems for you.

Are there any benefits for women from intermittent fasting?

Based on what we observe, if the body sees it as a major stressor, intermittent fasting potentially affects reproductive health.

Your overall health and fitness are affected by something that affects your reproductive health.

And if you're not planning on having any biological children.

However, intermittent protocols of fasting differ, with some being far more severe than others. And variables such as your age, your dietary status, the amount of time you are fasting, and other stressors in your life, including exercise, are also likely to be important.

THE PERFECT WOMEN'S INTERMITTENT FASTING SCHEDULE

There are several ways of dipping your toe in if you ever want to try intermittent fasting.

Given how much remains unknown, instead of diving into advanced intermittent fasting, a cautious approach is probably safer.

For a few days, you could start by keeping a food journal. Get a sense of what you eat, how much, and how often you eat it.

Do you eat late at night and have snacks during the day? Do your servings, or do you prefer lighter meals, seem to be large and fill you up? Do you get protein for every meal? Huh? Veggies?

"You should experiment with intermittent fasting "lite" once you have some more knowledge of your baseline. Here are a few ways to do that.

Start by stretching the interval between eating. What happens when you stop, if you normally snack between meals? Are you feeling greedy, dizzy, and mad? Does starvation ebb and flow? Do you feel totally fine?

Try to extend the time between your last meal in the evening and the next morning for your first meal. For instance, if you usually eat your last meal at 8 p.m. and then eat breakfast at 7 a.m. (11 a.m. fasting), try to eat your last meal at 6 p.m. and eat breakfast at 8 or 10 a.m. a little later (fasting 14-16 hours).

As you attempt these experiments, continue to physically check-in with yourself:

Although you may be a little bit more uncomfortable than usual, is the hunger manageable overall? Or do you notice that even now?

- Are you more or less reactive when stress spikes?

- What is your sleep like?

- Your drive for sex?

- Your levels of energy?

- Your workout performance?

Often check in with your thoughts about food and your body:

- Do you feel embarrassed or ashamed if you have to break early on the fast?

- Do you feel deprived and so overeat when it is permissible to eat?

- Do you feel hypercritical about the shape of your body or tie sentiments of meaning to how fine you are IF-ing?

Track yourself with curiosity, compassion, and integrity.

If you're feeling mentally sharp, energetic, and all systems are normal, proceed with a gentle intermittent fasting method, or try extending the fasting window a little further.

When to avoid intermittent fasting

If you're feeling obsessive, unhinged, and chronically lethargic, ease off.

Stop intermittent fasting if:

- your menstrual cycle ceases or becomes erratic

- you have trouble falling asleep or staying asleep

- your hair starts falling out more than normal

- you start to grow dry skin or acne

- you're finding you don't recover from workouts as quickly

- your injuries are slow to heal, or you get any bug going around

- Declines in the stress tolerance

- Your mood begins to swing.

- Your heart begins to go pitter-patter oddly.

- Your interest in romance fizzles (and when it does, your lady parts stop appreciating it),

- Your digestion slows down considerably,

- It still seems like you feel cold.

- Add some snacks, and/or reduce to 12 hours or less your nightly fasting time.

Don't get caught up in doing it right." There are many ways to change bodies, as we've learned from coaching more than 100,000 clients, and none of those approaches requires you to be flawless.

What to do if it isn't for you to fast

When you think intermittent fasting isn't a good fit, how do you get in shape and lose weight?

Know the fundamentals of outstanding eating.

Fasting or not, concentrating on meal quality does not go wrong: prioritize lean proteins, colourful vegetables, and fruits, healthy fats, quality carbohydrates. Crowd out snacks, caloric drinks, and foods that are refined. Cook and eat food in its entirety. Regularly workout. Remain consistent.

(And if you want any help doing all this, recruit a coach.)

By far, the best things you can do for your health and wellbeing are these simple fundamentals.

Sure, it may be common for intermittent fasting. And maybe it's a great fitness and health help for your brother or your boyfriend or your husband or even your dad.

Yet women are different than men, and there are different needs in our bodies.

Best Types Of Intermittent Fasting For Women

There is no one-size-fits-all strategy when it comes to dieting. For intermittent fasting, this often applies.

Women should usually take a more relaxed approach to fast than men.

This can include shorter periods of fasting, fewer days of fasting, and/or a limited amount of calories expended on days of fasting.

Here are some of the best kinds of women's intermittent fasting:

Crescendo Method: Fasting for two or three days a week for 12-16 hours. Fasting days in the week should be non-consecutive and uniformly spaced (for example, Monday, Wednesday, and Friday).

Eat-stop-eat (also referred to as the 24-hour protocol): Once or twice a week, a complete 24-hour fast: (maximum of two times a week for women). Start with fasting for 14-16 hours and build up gradually.

The 5:2 diet (also called "The Fast Diet"): Limit

calories for two days a week to 25 % of your usual consumption (about 500 calories) and consume the remaining five days "normally." Between fasting days, allow one day.

Alternate-Day Fasting Modified: Fasting every other day while eating on non-fasting days "normally." On a fasting day, you can eat 20-25% of your usual calorie consumption (about 500 calories).

The 16/8 Method (also referred to as the "Leangains method"): 16 hours a day fasting and eating all calories within an 8-hour window. It is recommended that women begin 14-hour fasts and gradually build up to 16 hours.

Whatever you choose, eating well during non-fasting times is still relevant. During the non-fasting times, if you consume many unhealthy, calorie-dense foods, you will not achieve the same weight loss and health benefits.

The right strategy at the end of the day is one that you can tolerate and maintain in the long term, which does not have any detrimental health effects.

CHAPTER 6

THE 12 MUST-KNOW TIPS FOR A HEALTHY AND EFFECTIVE FASTING DIET.

1. Ease yourself into your new meal schedule.

Accarding to Michal Hertz, RD, a dietitian in New York City, while it might be tempting to jump right into your new eating routine (the initial excitement is real), doing so can be difficult and leave you with increased hunger and discomfort. Instead, she recommends starting slowly during the first week by, say, doing two to three days of IF and then "gradually increasing week to week." Taking things slow is not just a great tip for fasting, but a great tip for life (just saying '). Taking things slow is a great tip for life.

2. Understand the distinction between having to eat and wanting to eat.

Once you hear your stomach growl, you may feel like there's no way you can get more hours without food through X. Tune in to the cue for hunger. "Ask yourself whether the hunger is actual hunger or boredom," "If you are bored, distract yourself with another task."

If you feel hungry but not weak or dizzy (which are signs, btw, that you should stop fasting ASAP), then sip a hot mint tea, as it is known that peppermint reduces appetite, or have water to help fill your stomach until your next meal, according to Savage.

Now, if for a while you've been trying IF and still feel extreme hunger between periods, then you need to think a little bit. During your eight-hour cycle, you need to add more nutrient- or calorie-dense foods or accept that this might not be the best plan for you. The addition of healthy fats such as almond butter, avocado, and coconut and olive oils, as well as proteins, during eating times, will help keep you happy and full longer.

3. Eat when necessary.

Technically, when following the 16:8 fasting method (perhaps the most common one), according to Hertz, extreme hunger and exhaustion do not occur. But if you feel lightheaded, listen up because the chances are that your body is trying to say something to you. You are likely to have low blood sugar and need to eat something, and that's all right, repeat after me.

By definition, fasting includes eliminating some, if not all, food, so don't beat yourself up with small, and smart, to break your fast! -Bites, bites. Hey, your best bet? As Savage suggests, go for a protein-rich snack such as one to two hard-boiled eggs or a few slices of turkey breast (to help stay in a ketogenic (fat-burning) state). You should then go back to fasting, that is, if you feel up to it, of course.

4. Hydrate

Even when you fast, drinking water and bevvies such as coffee and tea (without milk) are not only permitted but are encouraged per Hertz, particularly in the case of H_2O.

She suggests setting reminders throughout the day to lap up plenty of liquids, particularly during fasting times. According to both Hertz and Savage, aim to fill in at least 2, if not 3, litres a day.

5. Slowly and slowly, break your fast.

You can feel like a human vacuum ready to suck up whatever's on your plate after going several hours without food. But according to studies, chowing down in minutes is not necessarily beneficial for your body or your waistline. Instead of encouraging your digestive system to completely process the food, Savage explains, you want to chew well and eat slowly. This will also encourage you to have a clearer understanding of your fullness to prevent overeating.

6. Stop eating excessively.

Just because you stopped fasting, on that note, doesn't mean that you can feast. You cannot only eat too much, it can leave you bloated and miserable, but it can also ruin the objectives of weight loss that probably led you in the first place to IF. To put it plainly, it's not necessarily how much is on your plate that will help you stay full longer, but what's on your plate. That takes me to the next tip for fasting...

7. Provide balanced meals.

Ultimately, providing a hearty blend of protein, fibre, healthy fats, and carbs will help you shed those pounds and keep away from intense hunger while fasting. Per Savage, a good example? Grilled chicken with half a small sweet potato and sautéed spinach with garlic and olive oil (you want about 4 to 6 oz of protein).

Hertz states that when it comes to fruits, you want to go for individuals with a low-glycemic index, which are slowly digested, absorbed, and metabolized, causing a lower and slower rise in blood glucose," A healthy blood-sugar level helps you resist cravings and is, therefore, necessary when it comes to falling lbs successfully.

8. Play around during various periods.

Although the 16:8 is often recommended by Hertz, she says to look at your overall lifestyle to see which fasting technique might suit best.

For example, if you always wake up early, Hertz recommends eating during the earlier hours, like 10 a.m. At 6 p.m., and then fast until 10 a.m. the next morning. Remember: The beauty of IF is that it suits you and your routine comfortably and flexibly.

According to Savage, another alternative is cutting

yourself off earlier and eating breakfast later every day to gradually increase your fasting power. For instance, "We all naturally fast once daily—while we sleep—so maybe you practice 'shutting down the kitchen' earlier." the kitchen at 9 p.m., and then don't eat again until breakfast at 8 a.m. For instance, close the kitchen at 9 p.m., and then do not eat again until breakfast at 8 a.m. That's a natural fast of 11 hours! If needed, she says, slowly shifts certain times out (e.g., the kitchen closes at 8 p.m., breakfast at 9 a.m.).

It imports this content from {embed-name}. On their website, you may be able to find the same content in another format, or you may be able to find more detail.

9. Steer clear of fasting for 24-hours.

Hertz states that both experts do not suggest fasting for a full day, as it can "lead to increased hunger, weakness, and increased food consumption—and thus, weight gain,"

If you aim to lose weight, it may be more helpful to consider your total caloric intake and focus on scaling down than toughing out a fast for a long time (especially if you're the type to binge after). Just take it from a study, which indicates that there are simply no further advantages than daily caloric restriction in fasting for 24 hours, Savage adds.

10. Customize your workout routine.

First thing first: If you do a fasting diet, you can most certainly exercise. But (!!) you want to be conscious of what sorts of movements you are making, and when. Savage says, "If you are choosing to exercise in a fasting state, I recommend exercising in the morning when you have the most energy,"

It's important to note that if you don't, in Savage's terms, "adequately fueling your muscles," then you're at a higher risk of injury. So on fasting mornings, you may want to try lower-impact exercises, such as yoga or steady-state cardio, and save the hard-core HIIT class for after you've eaten.

11. Keep track of your journey.

Believe it or not, it will assist you with your fasting diet to maintain a food log. Journal of food for fasting?! Yup, you heard that correctly. Although you might not chronicle as many foods, it will allow you to measure your progress by actively jotting down information such as any feelings and symptoms (hunger level, and fatigue, etc. that come up throughout IF,

Although you might not chronicle as many foods, it will allow you to measure your progress by actively jotting down information such as any feelings and symptoms (hunger level, and fatigue, etc. that come up throughout IF,

Is. Crucial. For symptoms such as dizziness, exhaustion, (unusual) irritability, headache, anxiety, and difficulty focusing, keep an eye out at all times. Consider breaking your fast if you encounter any of these. "These are signs that the body is going into starvation mode and may need nourishment," And if you start feeling colder than usual, she says, that's even more of a warning to stop fasting. Be patient.

Your body will probably take time to get used to fasting, and you may feel hungrier and weaker than normal. So don't freak out if you have a week or so of these (less serious) sensations. However, if these complications last longer and suffer symptoms such as that above dizziness, Savage advises that you dismiss the diet and try something else to help you achieve your goals. It's not worth getting sick for any amount of pounds-trust.

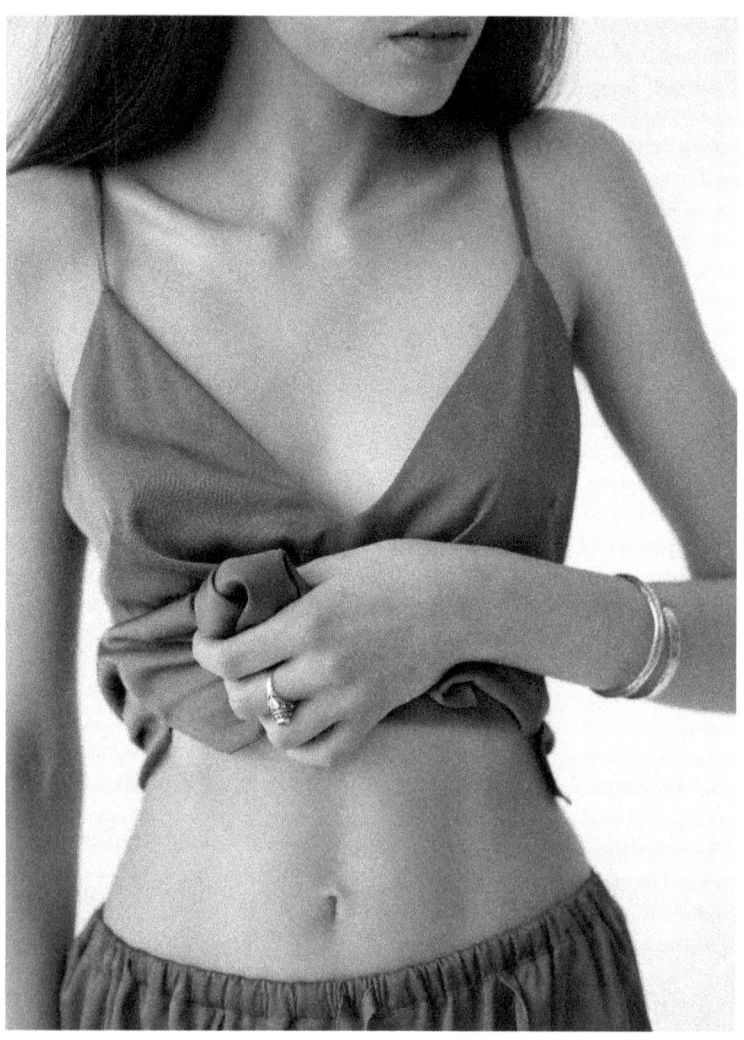

THE BEST EXERCISE ROUTINE FOR LONGEVITY

Here is the routine to optimize longevity that Longo recommends:

Walk fast every day for an hour

This need not happen all at once. For instance, if the train station is a 15-minute walk from your home, you do that every way you go, that's 30 minutes. Then you should select a coffee shop that is a 15-minute walk from your office and visit it every day. Those may not be your exact situations, but you get the concept of discovering walkable areas and going there every day. Walk everywhere, including faraway places on the weekend-do your best to leave your car all weekend long in the garage or driveway.

Practice 2.5 to 5 hours a week of aerobic exercise

Running, cycling or swimming are great choices, but it's not important what form of exercise you prefer. The trick is to work your body to the point of sweating and rapid breathing. Using a stationary bike and a road bike (go outdoors when the weather permits, otherwise ride indoors) is an easy way to meet this exercise threshold and make a point of cycling every other day for 30-40 minutes, and a total of 2 hours on the weekend.

To strengthen all muscles, use weight training or weight-free exercises to

This can be the classic workout routine, but when you take the stairs instead of the elevator (Longo suggests always taking the stairs!), walk instead of driving, grow food in your garden instead of buying it and do physical work around the house instead of hiring someone to do it, your muscles also become stronger. Consume at least 30 grams protein in a single meal within 1-2 hours to optimize muscle development while you participate in a tough weight training session.

Research reveals that much of the beneficial impacts are caused by the first 2.5 hours, in terms of how long you can exercise every week. A major Australian study of over 200,000 people aged 45-75, for instance, showed that those who exercised at least 2.5 hours per week at moderate to intense levels) had a 47 % reduction in overall mortality. Going up to 5 hours a week contributed to a mortality reduction of 54 %. The chance of dying dropped by another 9% by ensuring at least some of the operation was in the vigorous category.

Another very large research involving more than 650,000 individuals in the U.S. and Europe found that mortality was decreased by 31% for individuals exercising at moderate intensity for at least 2.5 hours a week (or for more than 75 minutes at vigorous intensity). The chance of dying was decreased by 37% by increasing the exercise total to 5 hours at moderate intensity (or 2.5 hours at intense levels).

Fast walking or slow jogging (faster than four mph), cycling (10–12 mph), or gardening are examples of moderate exercise. Climbing stairs or climbing, cycling (more than 12 mph), playing soccer, or jogging are physical exercise examples (faster than six mph).

There is, therefore, certainly some extra benefit of up to 5 hours of exercise every week, with some of the exercise being in the vigorous range. But after 2.5 hours, there are declining returns, and by going far past the 5-hour limit per week, you want to stop overworking your body. Over-exercising can cause damage to your knees, hips, and joints over time. Because of over-taxing, you don't want your body to break down prematurely.

My routine involves a casual run of 30 minutes in the morning, about five days per week. Thus, thanks to my morning run, I get 2.5 hours of moderate exercise per week. Then I add some vigorous exercise by playing squash for about 2 hours every week (I play twice a week, for an hour each time). In general, I'd say that I get about 4.5 total hours of workout per week.

And then I make a point of taking the stairs at all times. For instance, I take the stairs up to my floor from the parking garage at my office, a total of 111 steps. Every morning, climbing those stairs invigorates me for the workday ahead. Having meetings throughout the day on other floors allows me to rack up even more flights of stairs.

I walk whenever possible on the weekend. For example, take today's (I am writing this on a Sunday). This morning, I played squash for an hour and walked to the club and back for 15 minutes each way. I'm writing this from a coffee shop now, which is a 15-minute walk from my house. When I return home, in addition to my one-hour squash session, I will have walked for a total of one hour. In a walkable environment, I place a high value on living!

In the field of strength training, my routine is the lightest. Every day, I do 145 pushups, but otherwise, I do not do any kind of weight training. Squash is a full-body exercise, but I would like to add some more upper body strength training to ensure that my muscles remain strong as I age.

I considered exercise regularly to be an effective performance enhancer, and now I know how to exercise to improve a healthier lifespan.

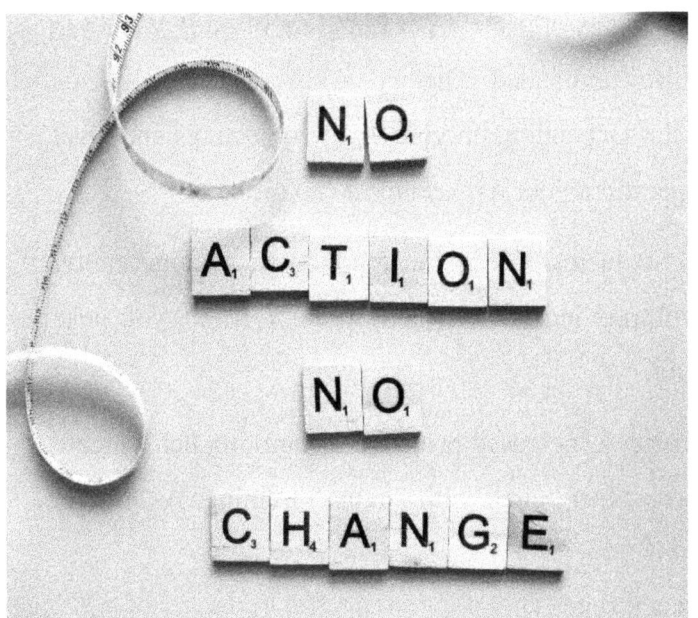

CHAPTER 7

INTERMITTENT FASTING FOOD LIST: HOW TO CHOOSE THE BEST FOODS

During intermittent fasting, feeding is more about being healthy than simply losing weight quickly. Thus, selecting nutrient-dense foods such as veggies, fruits, lean proteins, and healthy fats is critically important.

The list of intermittent fasting foods should include:

1. PROTEIN

0.8 grams of protein per kilogram of body weight is the Recommended Dietary Allowance (RDA) for protein. Depending on your health objectives and level of operation, your requirements can differ.

By reducing energy consumption, increasing satiety, and improving metabolism, protein helps you lose weight.

Besides, increased protein consumption helps create muscle when paired with strength training. As muscle burns more calories than fat, having more muscle in the body naturally increases the metabolism.

A recent study indicates that in healthy men, having more muscle in your legs will help reduce the development of belly fat.

The IF food list for protein include:

- Poultry and fish

- Seafood

- Eggs

- Dairy products such as yoghurt, milk, and cheese

- Beans and legumes

- Soy

- Seeds and nuts

- Whole grains

2. CARBS

45 to 65 per cent of the daily calories should come from carbohydrates, according to the Dietary Recommendations for Americans (carbs).

Carbs are the main source of your body's nutrition.

The other two are fat and protein. Carbs come in different ways. Sugar, carbohydrate, and starch are the most notable among them.

Carbs for causing weight gain also get a poor rap. Not all carbohydrates, however, are produced equally and are not necessarily fattening. The type and amount of carbs you eat depends on whether or not you can gain weight.

Make sure that foods high in fibre and starch but low in sugar are selected.

A 2015 study indicates that consuming 30 grams of fibre every day will lead to weight loss, glucose levels improving, and blood pressure decreasing.

It isn't an uphill struggle to get 30 grams of fibre from your diet. By consuming a basic egg sandwich, Mediterranean barley with chickpeas, peanut butter apple, and enchiladas with chicken and black peas, you will get them.

The IF food list for carbs include:

- Sweet potatoes
- Quinoa

- Oats

- Beetroots

- Brown rice

- Mangoes

- Apples

- Berries

- Bananas

- Kidney beans

- Pears

- Carrots

- Broccoli

- Brussels sprouts

- Avocado

- Almonds

- Chickpeas

- Chia seeds

3. FATS

Fats should contribute 20 per cent to 35 per cent of your daily calories, according to the 2015-2020 Dietary Recommendations for Americans. Most significantly, saturated fat does not account for more than 10% of daily calories.

Fats, depending on the form, maybe good, poor, or simply in-between.

Trans fats, for example, increase inflammation, decrease "good cholesterol levels and increase "bad cholesterol levels. They are found in fruit and baked goods that are fried.

Saturated fats can raise the risk of heart disease. Expert views on this, however, vary. Eating them in moderation is wise. High levels of saturated fats are present in red meat, whole milk, coconut oil, and baked goods.

The monounsaturated and polyunsaturated fats provide healthy fats. These fats can reduce the risk of heart disease, decrease blood pressure, and decrease fat levels in the blood.

The rich sources of these fats include olive oil,

peanut oil, canola oil, safflower oil, sunflower oil, and soybean oil.

The IF food list for fats include:

- Avocados

- Cheese

- Nuts

- Whole eggs

- Dark chocolate

- Chia seeds

- Fatty fish

- Full-fat yoghurt

- Extra virgin olive oil (EVOO)

4. For a HEALTHY GUT

An increasing body of evidence suggests that the secret to your overall wellbeing is your intestinal health. Your intestine has billions of bacteria known as microbiota in its home.

These bacteria impair your gut health, digestion, and

mental health. In many chronic disorders, they can also play a critical role.

Therefore, particularly when you are fasting intermittently, you should take care of those tiny bugs in your stomach.

The intermittent fasting food list for a healthy gut include:

- All vegetables
- Kefir
- Fermented vegetables
- Kimchi
- Miso
- Sauerkraut
- Kombucha
- Tempeh

These foods will also help you lose weight, in addition to keeping your gut safe by:

- Reducing fat absorption from the gut.

- Increasing the excretion via stools of ingested fat.

- Reducing the consumption of calories.

5. HYDRATION

The daily fluid requirement, according to the National Academies of Sciences, Engineering and Medicine, is:

About 3.7 litres (15.5 cups) for men.

About 2.7 litres (11.5 cups) for women.

Fluids include water, as well as water-containing foods and beverages.

During intermittent fasting, remaining hydrated is important for your health. Headaches, extreme tiredness and dizziness may be caused by dehydration. Dehydration can make these side effects of fasting worse or even extreme if you are still dealing with them.

The intermittent fasting food list for hydration include:

- Water

- Black coffee or tea

- Sparkling water

- Watermelon

- Cantaloupe

- Peaches

- Strawberries

- Oranges

- Lettuce

- Cucumber

- Skim milk

- Celery

- Plain yoghurt

- Tomatoes

Interestingly, drinking a lot of water will help with weight loss as well. A study reviewed in 2016 reports that proper hydration will help you lose weight through:

Decreasing appetite or consumption of food.

Rising burning of fat.

FOR FATS (75% OF YOUR DAILY CALORIES)

- Nuts

- Cheese

- Avocados

- Whole eggs

- Dark chocolate

- Chia seeds

- Extra virgin olive oil (EVOO)

- Fatty fish

- Full-fat yoghurt

FOR PROTEIN (20% OF YOUR DAILY CALORIES)

- Eggs

- Poultry and fish

- Seafood

- Seeds and nuts

- Dairy products such as yoghurt, milk, and cheese

- Soy

- Beans and legumes

- Whole grains

FOR CARBS (5% OF YOUR DAILY CALORIES)

- Beetroots

- Sweet potatoes

- Quinoa

- Brown rice

- Oats

The food list for intermittent fasting vegetarian diet includes:

FOR PROTEIN

- Seeds and nuts

- Dairy products such as yoghurt, milk, and cheese

- Beans and legumes

- Whole grains

- Soy

FOR CARBS

- Beetroots

- Sweet potatoes

- Quinoa

- Brown rice

- Bananas

- Oats

- Mangoes

- Apples

- Kidney beans

- Pears

- Berries

- Carrots

- Broccoli

- Brussels sprouts

- Avocado

- Almonds

- Chickpeas

- Chia seeds

FOR FATS

- Nuts

- Cheese

- Avocados

- Chia seeds

- Full-fat yoghurt

- Dark chocolate

- Extra virgin olive oil (EVOO)

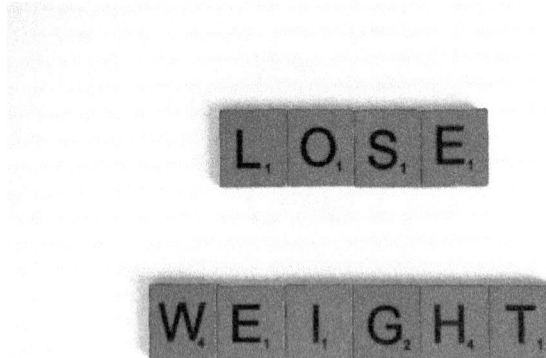

CONCLUSION

We cannot deny it: Time passes, and it changes our bodies. Our day-to-day wellbeing is like the weather, kind of. The cold comes and goes, like sunny days or storms going by, as do sniffles, pains and aches, blisters, and pimples. Our overall health is more like the environment, though. It's an aggregation of several different variables - biology, opportunity, and lifestyle choices we make - and in the long run, it has a larger effect on our lives.

The 50s means menopause for most women. But it just isn't a pause at all. Menopause looks more like a transition. Your levels of hormones move and change, and your body moves into a new state of equilibrium out of its childbearing years. But many women go through the often roller-coaster-like effects of menopause before achieving that equilibrium. You may experience hot flashes and night sweats during the time leading up to menopause, upset sleep and stress, mood swings, irritability, or depression.

As the hormone estrogen levels in your body decrease, you can also note other changes. Reduced vaginal lubrication can make it difficult, even painful, to have sexual intercourse and increase your risk of urinary and vaginal infections. Estrogen dips also cause the bone density to be lost - putting you at risk of osteoporosis - and have been associated with a gain in belly fat.

Belly fat can increase your risk of heart disease, diabetes, and cancer. You might need to bump up your exercises and lower your calorie intake to lose this weight. During this decade, your risk of colorectal cancer rises, so screening becomes important.

Poor pelvic muscles can play a role In urination problems like incontinence, and a condition called pelvic prolapse is to blame in some women. More prone are women who are obese or have had children. Excess weight can also put a woman at greater risk of developing uterine fibroids, which are non-cancerous tumours that grow but frequently shrink after they develop in the years before and during menopause. Heavy bleeding, pain during intercourse, frequent urination, and feelings of pelvic fullness are signs of fibroids.

Feeding an appetite for 50-something? Your changing body may need fewer calories as you move through menopause. At the same time, you can cope with decreased metabolism and become more susceptible to belly fat. Move high-fat foods to lower-fat alternatives and split them into leaner protein sources, such as chicken, fish, beans, or quinoa. Increasing your fruit and vegetable intake and encouraging healthy cholesterol and digestion with plenty of fibre gives your body an antioxidant gain.

KETO DIET FOR WOMEN OVER 50

The Winning Formula To Lose Weight and Increase Longevity + 30-Day Keto Meal Plan

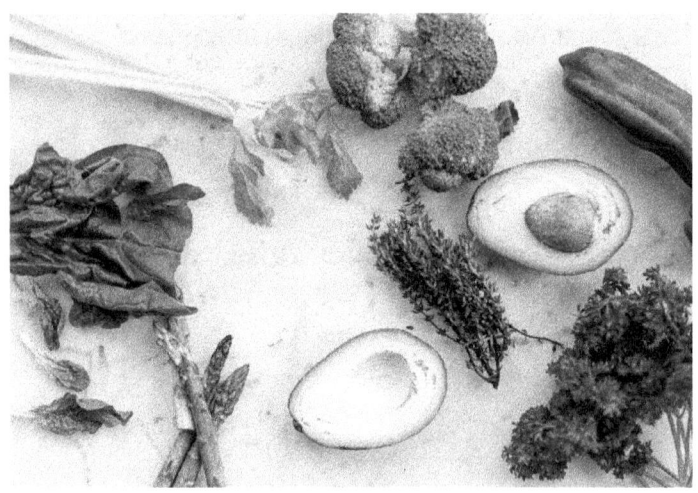

By

Stella Waters

inattention or otherwise, by any usage or abuse of any policies, processes, or directions contained within is the solitary and utter responsibility of the recipient reader. Under no circumstances will any legal responsibility or blame be held against the publisher for any reparation, damages, or monetary loss due to the information herein, either directly or indirectly.

Respective authors own all copyrights not held by the publisher.

The information herein is offered for informational purposes solely, and is universal as so. The presentation of the information is without contract or any type of guarantee assurance.

The trademarks that are used are without any consent, and the publication of the trademark is without permission or backing by the trademark owner. All trademarks and brands within this book are for clarifying purposes only and are the owned by the owners themselves, not affiliated with this document.

CHAPTER 1
THE KETO DIET

In particular, a ketogenic diet can be useful for losing weight without appetite and improving type 2 diabetes.

It is usually a diet that allows the body to discharge ketones into the bloodstream. As the body's main source of energy, most cells tend to use glucose, which originates from sugars. We begin to divide the extracted fat into particles called ketone bodies without circulating glucose from food (the procedure is called ketosis). Most cells can use ketone bodies to produce energy when you enter ketosis before we start eating carbohydrates again. As a rule, the transition from using circular glucose to separating put away fat as an energy source takes place more than two to four days of eating less than 20 to 50 grams of carbohydrates per day. Know, this is an incredibly individualized technique, and to begin supplying enough ketones, a few individuals need an increasingly restricted diet.

A ketogenic diet is rich in proteins and fats as it includes sugars. A variety of foods, eggs, treated meats, margarine, oils, sausages, cheeses, fish, nuts, seeds, and fibrous vegetables are frequently added. Since it is so prohibitive, when time progresses, it is exceedingly difficult to execute. At any point, carbohydrates regularly account for half of the popular American diet. One of the key reactions of this diet is that with not enough vegetables, many people would, in general, consume an abundance of protein and low-quality fats from processed foods. Since this diet could decrease their condition, patients with kidney sickness should be mindful. Also, in the first instance, a few patients will feel exhausted, while others may have nausea, constipation, awful breath, and trouble with sleep.

THE WAY KETO WORKS

The explanation for the ketogenic weight reduction diet is that if you deny the glucose community, the primary source of energy for all body cells obtained by consuming carbohydrate foods, an elective fuel called ketones is produced from the removal of fat (along these lines, the expression "keto"- genic). The mind gracefully asks for 120 grams a day for the most glucose in a routine, since it can't store glucose. The body first takes glucose away from the liver during fasting, or when virtually no food is ingested, and momentarily divides the muscle to release glucose. Blood levels of a hormone called insulin drop as this to go on for 3 to 4 days and storing away glucose is completely exhausted, and the body starts using fat as its essential fuel. Ketone bodies are made of fat in the liver and can be used without glucose.

This is called ketosis, at the point where ketone bodies amass the blood. During fasting cycles (e.g., sleeping for the moment) and demanding behaviour, healthy people, usually experience mild ketosis. Ketogenic diet proponents say that if the diet is followed carefully, there will be no dangerous blood levels of ketones (known as 'ketoacidosis') because the brain will use ketones for food and healthy people can produce enough insulin to avoid the production of excessive ketones. How rapid ketosis occurs and the amount of ketone bodies released in the blood varies from person to person and depends on components such as the metabolic rate of muscle-to-fat ratio and rest.

A variety of useful benefits are provided by selecting a ketogenic diet for diabetes control.

Research indicates that being in a dietary ketosis state substantially contributes to substantial changes in the regulation of blood glucose and weight loss.

Other common advantages include:

- Improvements in insulin sensitivity

- Reduced dependence on medication

- Usually improvements in cholesterol levels

- Lower blood pressure

We discuss the science behind the ketogenic diet in this book and how it works to provide all of these multiple benefits.

CHAPTER 2
UNDERSTANDING KETOSIS

What is ketosis?

K etosis is a metabolic condition where the bulk of the body's fuel is generated by fat.

It occurs when there is insufficient access to glucose (blood sugar), which is the body's preferred source of fuel for many cells.

Most generally, ketosis is associated with ketogenic and very low-carb diets. This also happens during pregnancy, fasting and malnutrition during childhood.

In general, to get into ketosis, individuals need to eat less than 50 grams of carbohydrates a day and sometimes as little as 20 grams a day.

It requires the absence of some food items, such as wheat, candy and soft drinks, from the diet. It is also essential to cut legumes, potatoes and berries.

Insulin levels of hormones decrease when consuming a very low-carb diet, and fatty acids are released from body fat stores in significant quantities.

Many of these fatty acids are transported to the liver and oxidized into ketones (or ketone bodies). With energy, these molecules will power the body.

In contrast to fatty acids, ketones can cross the blood-brain barrier and provide energy for the brain in the absence of glucose.

Ketosis is a metabolic disorder where the key sources of energy for the body and brain are ketones. This happens when there is a very low intake of carb and insulin content.

Ketones Supply Brain Energy

It is a common misconception that the brain doesn't work without dietary carbohydrates.

There is a real need for glucose, and there are other cells in the brain that can only use glucose as fuel.

However, ketones for energy, such as hunger or low carbohydrate diets, can also be used by a large part of your brain.

In fact, after just three days of starvation, the brain

obtains 25 % of its energy from ketones. During long-term hunger, this number increases to around 60 %.

Your body will then use protein to create a small amount of glucose that the brain still needs during ketosis.

Gluconeogenesis is known as the loop.

Ketosis and gluconeogenesis are capable of fulfilling the brain's energy needs well.

You will find more detail about ketogenic diets, and the brain here How low-carb and ketogenic diets enhance the safety of the brain.

If there's not enough glucose in the brain, then ketones can be used for energy. Protein can supply the limited amount of glucose it still needs.

Ketosis is NOT equivalent to ketoacidosis.

There is also a misunderstanding about ketosis and ketoacidosis.

While ketosis is part of normal metabolism, ketoacidosis is a hazardous metabolic disorder that can be lethal if left untreated.

Chronically elevated levels of glucose (blood sugar) and ketones join the bloodstream during ketoacidosis.

When this occurs, the blood becomes acidic, which is seriously dangerous.

In most cases, ketoacidosis is associated with uncontrolled type 1 diabetes. In individuals with type 2 diabetes, this may also happen, although this is less common.

Extreme alcohol abuse, however, may cause ketoacidosis,

Ketosis is a natural metabolic condition, and in uncontrolled type 1 diabetes, ketoacidosis is the most commonly observed serious medical disorder.

Impact on Epilepsy Symptoms

Epilepsy is a disease of the brain characterized by frequent seizures.

It is a very prevalent neurological disorder that affects approximately 70 million individuals worldwide.

In most patients, anti-seizure medications can help

treat seizures. Nevertheless, when using these drugs, about 30 % of patients still have seizures.

The ketogenic diet was introduced in people who did not respond to drug treatment as a remedy for epilepsy in the early 1920s.

It has been used mostly in children, with major advantages shown by some studies. Most epileptic children have recorded major reductions in seizures on a ketogenic diet, and some have even seen complete remission.

Ketogenic diets, particularly in children with epilepsy who do not respond to traditional treatment, can effectively reduce epileptic seizures.

Impact on Losing Weight

A ketogenic diet is a common weight loss diet that is well supported by science.

Indeed several studies have shown that, compared with low-fat diets, ketogenic diets contribute to much greater weight loss.

One study recorded 2.2 times greater weight loss for individuals on a ketogenic diet than those on a low-fat, calorie-restricted diet.

What's more, it seems like a ketogenic diet linked to ketosis makes people feel less hungry and more burdened. For this reason, on this diet, calories are typically not supposed to be counted.

Research suggests that, compared to low-fat diets, ketogenic diets contribute to greater weight loss. Humans, therefore, feel less hungry and more full.

Other Health Advantages of Ketosis

Ketosis and diets that are ketogenic may also have possible therapeutic effects. They're being tested today as a treatment for a wide variety of circumstances.

- Heart disease: reducing carbohydrate ketosis can increase risk factors for heart disease, such as triglycerides in the blood, total cholesterol and HDL cholesterol.

- Type 2 diabetes: The diet may increase insulin sensitivity by up to 75 %, and diabetes drugs may be minimized or even avoided by some diabetics.

- Metabolic syndrome: all the main signs of

metabolic syndrome, including elevated triglycerides, excess belly fat and high blood pressure, can be improved by ketogenic diets;

- Alzheimer's disease: Alzheimer's patients can benefit from a ketogenic diet.

- Cancer: Some studies indicate that in cancer treatment, ketogenic diets can be successful, possibly by helping to "starve" glucose cells.

- Parkinson's disease: A small study revealed that after 28 days on the ketogenic diet, Parkinson's symptoms improved.

- Acne: There is some evidence that this diet may reduce acne incidence and growth.

A variety of medical conditions, including metabolic syndrome, type 2 diabetes and Alzheimer's disease, can be improved by ketosis and ketogenic diets.

Is ketosis going to have any harmful health effects?

There are a few potential side effects you can experience from ketosis and ketogenic diets.

These include nausea, fatigue, constipation, high cholesterol, and bad breath.

However, most of the symptoms are mild and will vanish in a couple of days or weeks.

On a diet, some kids with epilepsy have also developed kidney stones.

And while extremely rare, there have been a few cases of women breastfeeding who are likely to develop ketoacidosis from a low-carb or ketogenic diet.

People who take blood sugar-lowering drugs should consult with a doctor before attempting a ketogenic diet, since the need for medication may be decreased by the diet.

Ketogenic diets also have poor nutrient content. It is a good idea to make sure you eat plenty of high-fibre low-carb vegetables for this reason.

With that being said, the well is normally safe for ketosis.

And it will not suit everyone. Some people will feel good and full of life in ketosis, while others will feel sad.

10 SIGNS THAT YOU ARE IN KETOSIS

Here are ten normal signs and symptoms of ketosis, both positive and negative.

1. Bad Breath

After getting to complete ketosis, individuals also experience bad breath.

This is usually a popular side effect. Most people report receiving a fruity scent as their breath takes on ketogenic diets and similar diets, such as the Atkins diet.

High levels of ketones are attributed to it. Acetone, a ketone in your urine and breath that exits the body, is the specific culprit.

Even though this breath may be less than optimal for your social life, it may be a good sign for your health.

To resolve the problem, most ketogenic dieters brush their teeth several times a day or use sugar-free gum.

Look for carbohydrates in the bottle, whether you use gum or other alternatives, such as sugar-free drinks. This can raise blood sugar levels and decrease levels of ketones.

Ketone acetone is partially extracted from your breath and can cause poor or fruity-smelling breath to be caused by a ketogenic diet.

2. Loss of weight

Alongside normal low-carb diets, ketogenic diets are highly effective for weight loss.

As dozens of weight loss studies have shown, you'll probably experience both short- and long-term weight loss when you switch to a ketogenic diet.

Quick weight-loss can occur within the first week. Although this is considered to be a fat loss by some people, it is mostly used for storing carbs and liquids.

After the initial rapid drop in water weight, you will begin to lose body fat slowly as long as you adhere to the diet and remain in a calorie deficit.

Fast weight loss generally occurs when a ketogenic diet is followed, and carbohydrates are severely restricted.

3. Improved Blood ketones

One of the hallmarks of a ketogenic diet is a decrease

in blood sugar levels and a rise in ketones.

You'll start consuming fat and ketones as the key sources of food when you work towards a ketogenic diet.

Using a specialized meter to measure your blood ketone concentrations is the most reliable and accurate method for measuring ketosis.

It tests your ketone levels by measuring the amount of beta-hydroxybutyrate (BHB) in your blood.

This is one of the ketones in the bloodstream that is most important.

According to some experts on the ketogenic diet, dietary ketosis is characterized as blood ketones ranging from 0.5–3.0 mmol / L.

Measuring ketones in your blood is the most efficient method of testing and is used in most scientific studies. However, the biggest drawback is that a slight pinprick involves drawing blood from your finger.

What's more, it could be costly for test kits. Most individuals perform just one test per week or every other week for that reason.

Checking the blood ketone levels with a scale is the most accurate way to determine whether you are in ketosis.

4. Increases ketones in urine or breath

Another way to monitor blood ketone levels is by using a breath analyser.

This tracks acetone, which during ketosis is one of the three primary ketones in your blood.

This gives you an idea of your body's ketone levels since more acetone leaves the body with nutrients when you are in ketosis.

The use of acetone breath analyzers is reasonably efficient but less accurate than the blood monitoring system used.

Special indicator strips to regularly measure the concentration of ketones in the urine are another effective strategy.

Ketone excretion through the urine is also measured and can be a simple and cheap way to test ketone levels every day. However, they aren't considered very accurate.

To test ketone levels, you may use a breath analyser or urine strips. However, they're not as accurate as a blood monitor.

5. The Suppression of Appetite

When following a ketogenic diet, most individuals experience reduced hunger.

The reasons for this are still under inquiry.

However, it has been suggested that this reduction in hunger may be due to increased protein and vegetable intake, along with changes to your body's starvation hormones.

To reduce your appetite, even the ketones themselves can affect your brain.

A ketogenic diet can decrease hunger and appetite dramatically. You might be in ketosis when you feel full and do not have to feed as much as before.

6. Heightened focus and energy

When they start a very low-carb diet first, people also experience brain fog, fatigue and feeling sick. It is referred to as low carb flu' or' keto flu.' However, long-term ketogenic dietitians also show enhanced concentration and strength.

If you start a low-carb diet, your body needs to change to eat more fat for fuel instead of carbs.

A large part of the brain starts to consume ketones rather than glucose once you get into ketosis. It may take a few days or weeks for you to get off properly.

A very potent source of fuel for your brain is ketones. They have also been studied in a medical environment to treat brain disorders and conditions like concussion and memory loss.

It comes as no surprise; therefore that long-term ketogenic dieters often report enhanced brain function and clarity.

It is also possible to remove carbs and can help regulate and maintain levels of blood sugar. This will enhance concentration further and improve brain activity.

Better brain activity and more stable energy levels are reported by most long-term ketogenic dieters, possibly due to the increase in ketones and healthy blood sugar levels.

7. Short-Term Fatigue

The initial switch to a ketogenic diet may be one of the biggest issues for new dietitians. Fatigue and weakness may include its reported side effects.

These also lead individuals before going into full ketosis to leave their diet and reap many of the long-term benefits.

These are normal side effects. Since the body has been running for many decades on a carb-heavy fuel system, it is forced to adapt to another system.

This transition, as you would expect, isn't happening immediately. Before you get into full ketosis, it usually takes 7-30 days.

During this round, you may want to take electrolyte supplements to reduce fatigue.

Due to the rapid decline in the body's water content and the removal of refined foods that may have added salt, electrolytes are also lost.

Try taking these supplements to get 2,000-4,000 mg

of sodium, 1,000 mg of potassium and 300 mg of magnesium per day.

You might suffer from exhaustion and low strength at first. This will pass if the body is conditioned to work on fat and ketones.

8. Short-term decreases in performance

As discussed above the removal of carbs will lead to general tiredness at first. This involves an initial decrease in performance during exercise.

It is mainly caused by the decrease in your muscles' glycogen stores, which provide the primary and most effective source of fuel for all forms of high-intensity exercise.

A lot of ketogenic dieters say that their performance returns to normal after several weeks. In certain types of ultra-endurance sports and operations, a ketogenic diet may also be useful.

Also, there are other benefits, namely an improved capacity to burn more fat during exercise.

One well-known study showed that compared to athletes who did not practice this diet, athletes who converted to a ketogenic diet burned up to 230 % more fat while exercising.

Although a ketogenic diet is unlikely to improve efficiency for professional athletes, once you are fat-adapted, it should be appropriate for general exercise and recreational sports.

Degradations in short-term performance can occur. However, they continue to develop once more after the initial adaptation process is over.

9. Digestive issues

A ketogenic diet normally requires a significant shift in the types of food you eat.

Initially, digestive problems such as constipation and diarrhoea are normal side effects.

After the transition period, some of these issues should subside, but it may be important to be aware of the different foods that may cause digestive problems.

Also, make sure that lots of good low-carb vegetables are eaten that are low in carbohydrates but have plenty of fibre in them as well.

Do not make a mistake, above all of eating a diet that lacks variety. This can increase your risk of digestive problems and deficiencies in nutrients.

You may experience digestive problems, like constipation or diarrhoea, when you first turn to a ketogenic diet.

10. Insomnia

One major problem with too many ketogenic dieters is sleep, especially when they first change their diet.

Most individuals experience sleeplessness or even waking up at night when they first increase their carbohydrates dramatically.

Nevertheless, it generally changes in a matter of weeks.

A lot of long-term ketogenic dieters say they sleep better than before after adapting to the diet.

CHAPTER 3

MENOPAUSE AND KETOGENIC DIET

What is the Change from Menopause?

While a woman technically enters menopause when she has gone 12 months without a menstrual cycle, perimenopause-related symptoms will begin much sooner, when hormonal changes begin. Furthermore, after this stage, they may last for several years, and new symptoms may arise during the first few years after menopause.

The average perimenopause onset age is 46, and it usually lasts for around seven years. However, between her mid-30s and mid-50s, a woman can begin perimenopause at any time, and the process may last from 4 to 14 years. She is considered postmenopausal on the day after a woman has gone 12 months without a menstrual cycle.

As many as 34 symptoms can occur during and after

the transition from menopause. The most prevalent ones include:

- Hot flashes and night sweats
- Weight gain, especially around the middle
- Insomnia
- Vaginal dryness
- Mood swings
- Fatigue
- Poor memory, i.e., "brain fog."

Interestingly, when some women learn that their symptoms during perimenopause are more severe, others say that after they are postmenopausal, their symptoms intensify.

Fluctuations of hormones and resistance to insulin during menopause

Follicle Stimulating Hormone (FSH) induces the release of an egg from one of her ovaries approximately every 28 days during a woman's reproductive years and stimulates ovarian development of estrogen. The follicle housing the egg releases progesterone after ovulation.

However, her ovaries contain fewer eggs and continue to produce less estrogen and progesterone when a woman reaches perimenopause. In response, the pituitary gland of the brain steps up its FSH production to increase the production of estrogen. Estrogen levels may fluctuate widely during this period, but they decrease gradually during a final couple of years before menopause.

Estrogen usually guides fat to be accumulated after puberty in the hip and thigh zone. This is why many, but not all, women during their reproductive years appear to gain weight in this field.

However, during menopause, when estrogen levels decline, fat storage moves to the abdomen. Excess visceral fat doesn't just affect your body and the way your clothes fit, unlike the subcutaneous fat contained in your hips and thighs. Insulin resistance, heart disease and other health issues are also closely related.

MENOPAUSE AND WEIGHT GAIN

In addition to the transition in fat distribution, during and after perimenopause, most women find that their weight increases by many pounds. This appears to be attributed to a mixture of variables.

Next, lower estrogen levels cause insulin resistance and higher blood insulin or hyperinsulinemia levels, which promote weight gain.

Furthermore, evidence indicates that in the early stages of perimenopause, levels of the "hunger hormone" ghrelin increase.

Also, low levels of estrogen during and after menopause can impair leptin and neuropeptide Y development, hormones that help regulate appetite and weight balance. Overeating and weight gain will result from the resulting increase in appetite and lack of satiety.

However, due to the hormonal changes previously mentioned, some women put on weight even though they don't eat more than normal during menopause.

Finally, the loss of muscle mass during menopause and the ageing process will slow down the metabolism, making it much simpler to put on weight.

LOW-CARB AND KETO MENOPAUSAL SYMPTOM DIETS

Managing Weight

There is a rising body of research that shows that low-carb and keto diets are very successful for weight loss.

A significant advantage of ketosis is appetite reduction, which could be partly attributed to lower levels of ghrelin.

Indeed a 2014 systematic review of 12 studies concluded that ketogenic diets decrease hunger and appetite. Also, the researchers identified a ketogenic diet as one that yielded fasting levels of β-hydroxybutyrate greater than or equal to 0.3 mMM. This is a very mild ketosis level that can be accomplished by most individuals by limiting the intake of net carb to 50 grams or less per day.

Anecdotally, before and after menopause, many women have reported losing weight by adopting a low-carb or keto diet.

However, while some studies on carb restriction have involved middle-aged and older women, there is relatively little research looking at the consequences of this way of eating in menopausal women alone.

A low-carb, paleo diet resulted in greater reductions in abdominal fat and triglycerides than women adopting a low-fat diet in a two-year randomized controlled trial (RCT) of 70 obese postmenopausal women.

In another RCT, either a calorie-restricted diet or a non-calorie-restricted diet initially supplying 20 grams of carb per day was followed by 50 overweight or obese middle-aged women who steadily increased by 10 grams per week over 12 weeks. The low-carb group saw a larger reduction in triglycerides and a greater increase in cholesterol ratios than the calorie-restricted group. In contrast, the two groups lost identical amounts of weight.

It is worth pointing out that while the low-carb community began consuming a keto diet, by the end of the study, they were no longer similar to ketosis at 140 grams of carb. This illustrates that weight loss doesn't need to adopt a very low carb strategy resulting in high ketone levels.

Clearly, in menopausal women, more high-quality research needs to be done on low-carb and keto diets. It is fair, however, that it will be very good for them to eat in a way that reduces insulin levels and helps regulate appetite.

THE SIDE EFFECTS OF TRANSITIONING TO KETO DIET

While the adverse effects associated with the ketogenic diet are usually less beneficial than those of anticonvulsant drugs used to treat epilepsy, there can be a range of negative effects in people adopting the diet.

Side Effects in the short term

At the beginning of therapy, many short-term side effects are most apparent, particularly when patients start the diet with an initial fast.

In this case, hypoglycemia is a common side effect, and visible signs can include:

- Excessive thirst

- Frequent urination

- Fatigue

- Hunger

- Confusion, anxiety and/or irritability

- Tachycardia

- Lightheadedness and shakiness

- Sweating and chills

Patients can also experience some constipation and low-grade acidosis also. When the diet is continued, these results appear to change, as the body adapts to the new diet and modifies how it produces energy.

Alteration in Blood Composition

There are numerous shifts in the blood composition of individuals adopting the ketogenic diet as a result of changes in food consumption and the body's adaptive mechanisms to cope with the decreased intake of carbohydrates.

Lipid and cholesterol levels in the blood, in particular, are typically higher than what is considered normal. About 60 % of patients have elevated lipid levels, and over 30 % have high cholesterol levels.

If these changes are profound and there is some concern about the child's health, for the particular patient, minor changes may be made to the diet. Saturated fat sources, for instance, can be substituted for polyunsaturated fats. In certain cases, the ketogenic ratio will need to be lowered, and the proportion of fat in the diet to carbohydrates and proteins reduced.

Long-lasting effects

Other adverse effects become more apparent and have a greater impact on individuals when the ketogenic diet is maintained for longer periods.

Kidney stones, also known as nephrolithiasis, are a common complication of the disorder in children after dieting, with around 5% of patients suffering from it. It is, however, treatable and it is recommended by the latest guidelines that the diet should continue. It is suspected that the development of kidney stones is related to hypocitraturia and hypercalciuria when acidosis induces demineralization of the bone. Also, low pH in the urine can promote crystal formation and, ultimately, kidney stones.

There is some evidence that potassium citrate supplementation decreases the occurrence of kidney stones since it binds to the bloodstream and reduces the amount of calcium. However, further research on this is needed.

Also, there is an increased risk of bone fractures in patients. This is due to the altered levels of growth factor 1-like insulin and the symptoms of acidosis. Acidosis results in bone erosion, weakening the bones and leaving them vulnerable to fractures.

Supplementation of vitamins and minerals is regularly given to patients following a ketogenic diet to treat these side effects. This usually involves supplements with multivitamins, calcium and vitamin D.

Adult Side Effects

The most common risks for adults following a ketogenic diet include loss of weight, constipation, and elevated cholesterol and triglyceride levels. Women can also encounter amenorrhea or other menstrual cycle disturbances.

WHERE TO START FOR WOMEN MORE THAN 50

Although keto is a simple diet, it's not always easy to make the transition from a high carb diet to consuming 50 grams or less of carbs per day.

Make your move to a low-carb keto diet smoother by following these guidelines.

1. Got a scheduled start date

Keto is different from other diets, so you can't immediately jump in without doing your homework.

Select a starting date and let yourself know about the low-carb diet's ins and outs.

Read all on what should be eaten and what should not be eaten. Spend this time collecting any low-carb tools that could be beneficial, such as meal plans and recipes.

Also, tell your family and friends that you are "going keto" and are about to change your diet.

Tell them to be patient and understand that you won't be eating bread, rice, pasta, etc., anytime.

2. Remove needless carbohydrates from your closets.

Just before you launch your keto diet, clean your kitchen cupboards and the refrigerator with any non-keto foods.

You may think that you can conquer the temptation and not eat it, but the truth is that you are more likely to break your diet if you have easy access to high-carb foods.

Do not make a mistake, however of eating all these foods. The slower and more complicated your transition to ketosis is going to be the more carbs you eat in the keto lead-up.

3. Use an App for food tracking

Successful keto diet suggests that the intake of carb is limited to 50 grams or less per day.

Using a food tracking app to do that effectively is the simplest, if not the only way.

Armed with your simple-to-use macro tracker, you

can fine-tune your meals to get the right intake of carbohydrates, protein and fat.

4. Assume the first two weeks are the worst,

It's not always easy to get keto in the first two weeks, in particular.

It takes time for your body to use all of its onboard carb stores and to turn to use ketones for energy instead.

Some individuals experience adverse side effects during this period, which are usually called keto flu.

While keto flu is not serious and does not attract, until your body reaches complete ketosis, you can feel unwell.

Symptoms of keto flu popular to all include:

1. Headaches

2. Nausea

3. Breastfeeding

4. Insomnia

5. fruity-smelling breath

6. Increased urination

7. Fatigue

8. Mood swings

9. Cravings

The good news is that these signs mean that your body is beginning to change from using carbohydrates to using energy ketones. You are well on the way to being a fat-consuming weapon. The signs will fade rapidly, and within 1-2 weeks, they will pass away entirely. Even after they've died, and unless you cheat on your diet, you can experience keto flu only once.

5. Don't cheat at all

By eating unhealthy foods, several diets allow you to take days off and even cheat from time to time. The keto diet is no diet like that! You will get kicked out of ketosis when you cheat on keto by eating carbs and need to go through another bout of keto flu to get back on track.

Don't be tempted to cheat on keto for a long story; it just isn't worth it. Using other kinds of therapies instead to reward your healthy eating habits. Going to the movies, or treating yourself to a beauty treatment or massage or purchasing a new workout outfit are nice choices. High carb nutritional treatments are not part of a ketogenic diet.

6. Consider using a few well-chosen additions

They will make it simpler for women over 50 years of age, but you don't have to use keto diet supplements. Contains: Nice choices

1. exogenous Ketones

Exogenous ketones are ketones from an alien source. Taking exogenous ketone supplements can keep your mind calm, provide you with energy, speed up fat burning, and can help relieve the symptoms of many of the keto flu. In capsules and as drink mixes, exogenous ketones can be contained.

2. medium-range Triglycerides

In short, MCTs transform these unique fats into ketones rapidly and easily. Increased fat burning and weight loss, less strength, and fewer symptoms of keto flu mean fewer ketones.

The MCT supplements are made from palm oil or

coconut oil. However, coconut oil is the safest option and is also the most environmentally friendly. MCTs are available as oils or in a powder form that is simple to blend.

3. Electrolyte

In your urine, electrolytes are minerals that are excreted and even lost as you sweat.

The keto diet increases urine production, and that may mean that these vital substances start running low on your body. Muscle cramps and headaches include symptoms of low electrolyte levels.

Electrolyte supplements replace the missing minerals and can help prevent the effects of some of the keto flu.

7. Treat keto as a way of life, not just a diet.

They just plan to follow it for a couple of weeks, as most people think of a new diet. They find that once they have lost some weight, they will struggle through it, and then they go back to their previous way of eating. Invariably, this results in weight loss accompanied by weight recovery, which experts call the yoyo diet.

You will get even better outcomes with keto if you

accept a low-carb diet as a lifestyle choice and not a short-term solution. Not only are you going to lose weight this way, but you're also going to keep it off for good.

Also, most of the benefits listed earlier in this article are only applicable if you have a low carb diet. If you break your diet, you will say goodbye to conditions like lower blood pressure, improved cardiovascular health, reduced inflammation, and better bone health.

In your 50s, Keto is great for weight loss, but it can also be so much more. On every aspect of your wellbeing, it can have a profound and substantial impact.

After a few weeks or months, don't throw away the advantages by hitting and leaving Keto. Instead, commit yourself to a low-carb diet for the long term. You're going to enjoy the outcome if you do.

What are Keto-Approved Foods?

WLose Weight On Keto for Women Over 50h While it's easy to assume that the keto diet is high in fat and low in carbs when you're in the supermarket aisle, it still seems a little more difficult.

LIST OF KETO-BASED FOODS FOR WOMEN OVER 50.

What Keto Foods to Eat

Meat: check for unprocessed meats because they have less or no) carbs added

Meat and seafood: skip the added carbs from breaded fish

Eggs: prepared, but the best you want,

Vegetables: those rising above the ground

Dairy: opt for high-fat milk; sugar has also been added to low-fat alternatives.

Nuts: a decent source of fat, but be careful not to consume too much.

Berries: in moderation concerning

What foods should not be consumed on Keto?

Sugar: the main thing that should be cut

Fruit: a little fruit is all right, but too much adds sugar to your diet,

Beer/Alcohol: so many sugars and carbohydrates

Starches: white bread, corn, potatoes, pasta

Your favourite foods by Keto-frying

Any of your favourite foods may be on the no-no list above, depending on what you enjoy eating.

It is still difficult to accept the drawbacks of a new diet. Keto-friendly plate

For our families and us, food and recipes can become so intimate that it's difficult to break away from them.

Fortunately, there are simple ways to make alternatives to your favourite foods so that they work into keto, or remain within a close window at least.

That means you can still have your pasta dishes and sandwiches in abundance! As a general rule, select carbohydrates that are most effective with a low glycemic index.

Bread: 20x fewer carbohydrates than standard bread

Pasta: recipe with two ingredients

Rice: Recipe with three ingredients

Oatmeal: a low-carb alternative for breakfast

For women over 50 years, is a Keto diet good?

Whether or not Keto is correct for you depends on a range of considerations.

A ketogenic diet can provide many benefits, especially for weight loss, assuming you do not suffer from health problems.

Eating a great mix of greens, lean meat, and unprocessed carbs is the most significant thing to note.

It is possible that sticking to whole foods is the most successful way to eat healthily, mostly because it is a sustainable strategy.

It is important to remember that a lot of research suggests that it is difficult to stick with ketogenic diets. For this reason, discovering a safe way of eating that works for you is the best advice.

A FULL FOOD GUIDE TO FOLLOW

Do you wonder what's going on in a keto diet and what's not? "It's so important to know what you're going to eat before you start and how to incorporate more fats into your diet, "It's so important to know what you're going to eat before you start and how to incorporate more fats into your diet. We requested some directives from her.

Proteins

Liberally: (That said, ketogenic diets are not high in protein; they focus on fat, so all of them should be moderately consumed.)

- Grass-fed beef
- Dark meat chicken
- Fish, especially fatty fish, like salmon

Occasionally:

- Proteins low in fat, such as skinless chicken breast and shrimp. These are nice to include in your keto diet, but instead of eating simple, add a sauce to the top for some fat.
- Bacon

Never:

- Cold cuts with added sugar
- Meat marinated in sugary sauces
- chicken nuggets or fish

Fat and Oil

Liberally:

- Coconut oil
- Avocado oil
- Butter
- Olive oil
- Heavy cream

Occasionally: (Limit your intake, which should be easy to do when avoiding packaged foods, often found in)

- Sunflower oil
- Safflower oil
- Corn oil

Never:

- Margarine
- Artificial trans fats

Fruits and Veggies

- Liberally:
- Celery
- Leafy greens, like spinach and arugula
- Asparagus
- Avocado

Occasionally: (These are all fantastic options, but certain carbs will still need to be counted.)

- Spaghetti squash
- Leeks
- Eggplant

Never:

- Potatoes
- Raisins
- Corn

Nuts and Seeds

Liberally:

- Almonds
- Walnuts
- chia seeds and Flaxseed

Occasionally:

- Cashews
- Unsweetened nut butter (peanut butter or almond)
- Pistachios

Never:

- Sweetened nut or seed butter
- Trail mixes with dried fruit
- Chocolate-covered nuts

Dairy Products

Liberally:

- Cheddar cheese
- Feta cheese
- Blue cheese

Occasionally:

- Full-fat plain Greek yoghurt
- Full-fat cottage cheese
- Full-fat ricotta cheese

Never:

- Milk
- Ice cream
- Sweetened nonfat yoghurt

Sweeteners

Liberally: Practice moderation with sweeteners.

Occasionally:

- Erythritol
- Stevia
- Xylitol

Never:

- Maple syrup
- Agave

- White and brown sugars
- Honey

Condiments and Sauces

Liberally:

- Guacamole
- Mayonnaise (no sugar added)
- Lemon butter sauce

Occasionally:

- Tomato sauce (with no added sugar)
- Raw garlic
- Balsamic vinegar

Never:

- Ketchup
- Honey mustard
- Barbecue sauce

Drinks

- Almond milk
- Water
- Plain tea
- Bone broth

Occasionally:

- Unsweetened carbonated water (bound even if you get overwhelmed by bubbles)
- Black coffee (watch caffeine consumption)
- Diet soda
- Zero-calorie drinks

Never:

- Lemonade
- Fruit juice
- Soda

Herbs and Spices

Liberally: (All herbs and spices work into a keto diet, but Mancinelli recommends measuring the carbs if you use significant amounts.)

- Salt (salt foods to taste)
- Pepper
- Thyme, paprika, cayenne, and oregano

Occasionally:

- Onion powder
- ground ginger
- Garlic powder

Never:

- In general, herbs and spices are fine to use in small amounts to add flavour to food.

Supplements

Consider taking:

- Multivitamin
- Fibre
- Optional: (This helps you produce ketones faster, but Mancinelli says she has no opinion on recommending that you accept them or not.)
- Exogenous ketones
- MCT oil

12. RESPONSIBLY USE SWEETENERS.

Cutting out sugar is not easy, but it is worth it! Weight loss is the motivator for many people looking at keto diet advice, but increased strength, concentration, attitude, and other "NSV's" (non-scale victories) turn out to be a nice surprise for others. So getting rid of those sugar cravings feels like being SO. BIGHT. Uh.

That doesn't mean saying goodbye to all of the sweets, though! You can then make plenty of dessert recipes that are keto compliant.

The secret to both of those is the keto-friendly sweeteners. Here are the ones that I would propose:

- Monk Fruit

- Allulose

- Erythritol

Also to help you choose from, you can see a list of sweeteners here and bookmark the conversion calculator here, so you know how much.

13. GET SUPPORT

Starting with a new way of eating is not easy, and you don't have to do it alone!

There are hundreds of thousands of us in the community waiting for you to contribute. We have people at all stages of the journey, and we would love to have you in our group, whether you need a beginner's keto spot or you're a more experienced keto-er looking for someone to get it.

14. PLAN ANY MEAL.

One of the biggest tips and tricks I can tell people about keto is that a game-changer is meal planning. A bag of chips, a candy bar, or a box of pasta on a high-carb diet can be easy to grab, but more preparation is needed to stick to a low-carb lifestyle.

And that is flawless! It's doable, and it's not going to take hours out of the day.

Whether it's planning like I'm doing for the week ahead, or just looking at the morning ahead, you should make your schedule. Some people will find it helpful to enter what you are going to eat in advance when you are using a monitoring app, so you can prepare accordingly.

Or you can only use my keto diet menu for beginners, so I can do it for you.

At least loosely-planning what you eat every day will save you time and money. But it can also be challenging and time-consuming to come up with the strategy to make sure it fits your macros, provides enough range and tastes good.

This is why I make a simple keto meal plan for beginners each week. To save time and money, we combine meal preparation, super-fast meals (which will feed even non-keto family members!), and sometimes leftovers. I have single-person or four-family options, so it can suit your life.

CHAPTER 4
KETO BENEFITS FOR WOMEN
OVER 5O

K eto is viewed mainly as a weight loss diet. Low-carb keto diets, however, provide some additional major advantages to women in their 50s. Those benefits are:

1. Body fat reduced

A lot of diets promise weight loss, but in certain situations, the weight is just water. Keto increases weight reduction and creates better results than most other diets. Keto also targets abdominal fat, appropriately referred to as visceral fat; in females, abdominal fat tends to increase to more than 50. Which raises the risk of heart disease, stroke, and cardiac arrest. The accumulation of abdominal fat is primarily attributed to improvements in menopause-associated hormones.

2. Increased immunity to insulin

Carbs are digested and converted to glucose. When you ingest carbohydrates, your body releases the hormone insulin to carry the glucose into your liver and muscles. However, with age, the body's insulin sensitivity decreases, and that means that glucose is more likely to be converted into and processed as fat, contributing to weight gain.

Low-carb diets improve insulin sensitivity. That implies that the few carbs you consume do not turn into fat. The improved insulin sensitivity also helps to monitor your blood glucose levels. Low levels of blood glucose are inextricably associated with better general health and a decreased risk of type 2 diabetes.

3. Improved function of the brain

Menopausal women often encounter concerns such as memory loss, mood swings, and problems with concentration. Depression and anxiety can also cause them to suffer. This is because during menopause, the levels of estrogen, the main female sex hormone, decrease, affecting the amount of glucose that enters the brain.

The Keto diet provides your brain with an alternate source of fuel: ketones. Your mind functions better on ketones, and it is much less common to have issues like mood swings and memory loss on a low-carb diet.

A reduced incidence of various neurological disorders, including Alzheimer's disease and Parkinson's disease, is also correlated with the keto diet, both of which are more common in people over 50 years old.

4. decreases Inflammation

The ageing process can be rough on your body. Menopausal women experience knee and hip pain in their 50s, as well as headaches and other forms of non-specific pain.

Keto is a high-fat diet, and some fats are good for relieving inflammation. To be part of your keto diet, nice anti-inflammatory fats include:

- Olive oil
- Oily fish, for example, sardines, tuna, and salmon
- Avocados and Oil Avocado

- Walnuts

By comparison, foods like refined grains, sugar and processed foods are all associated with increased inflammation. Foods like that are not part of the keto diet.

5. Blood lipid profile improved

In their 50s, most females experience elevated levels of triglycerides and "poor" LDL cholesterol.

Here's a recipe for a heart attack.

While high in fat, it has been shown that low carb diets lower triglycerides and LDL cholesterol while increasing the levels of "good" HDL cholesterol.

Improved cardiovascular health and a decreased risk of heart disease are associated with these improvements.

6. Reduced blood pressure

Females appear to experience lower blood pressure than males. That will change as you reach your 50s, however, and menopause starts to take hold.

A host of serious health complications, including heart failure, stroke, and kidney disease, are associated with high blood pressure. The low-carb keto diet improves blood pressure control.

7. Elevated density of bone

Older women are vulnerable to bone loss and if left unchecked, may develop osteoporosis. This is a medical condition characterized by fragile bones that are fracture-prone.

Keto removes nutrients which are capable of interfering with calcium absorption. Keto, along with lots of leafy green vegetables that are naturally high in calcium, can help improve both bone strength and density.

8. Less muscle loss

In their fifties, women tend to lose their muscles more easily than in their twenties, thirties and forties. Muscle loss decreases the metabolic rate, leading to weight gain and making weight loss more difficult.

Your strength would also be impaired by muscle loss, making daily tasks more challenging and tiring.

A ketogenic diet allows moderate amounts of protein to be eaten, and protein is essential for the muscles to persevere. The protein comprises amino acids, and amino acids are the building blocks of muscle tissue.

Keto, both for weight loss and health improvement, can be very effective for women in their 50s.

Going keto means cutting out and replacing all the unhealthy foods we know with foods that are rich in beneficial nutrients.

In short, Keto is not only a diet for overweight people; it is a diet for anybody who wants to lead a healthier, longer life!

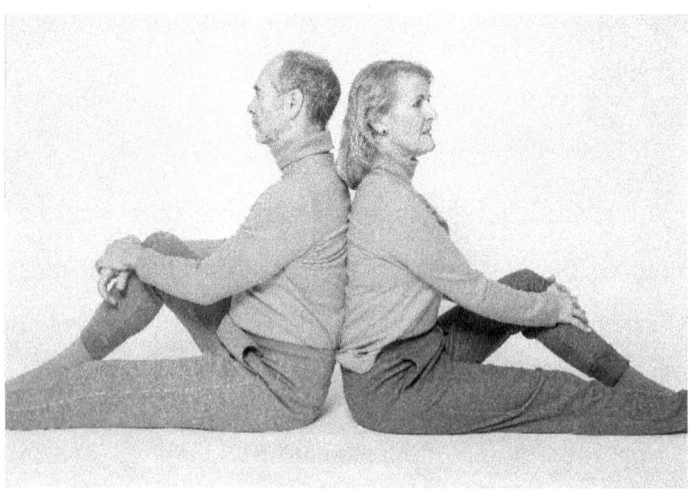

CHAPTER 5
30-DAY KETO DIET MEAL PLAN

WEEK 1

Day 1

Breakfast: Chorizo Breakfast Bake

Lunch: Sesame Pork Lettuce Wraps

Dinner: Avocado Lime Salmon

Total macros: Calories: 1,520, Fat: 109g, Protein: 110g, Net Carbs: 16g

Day 2

Breakfast: Leftover Chorizo Breakfast Bake with 3 Slices Thick-Cut Bacon

Lunch: Spiced Pumpkin Soup

Dinner: Leftover Avocado Lime Salmon

Total macros: Calories: 1,570, Fat: 124g, Protein: 92g, Net Carbs: 16g

Day 3

Breakfast: Baked Eggs in Avocado

Lunch: Easy Beef Curry

Dinner: Rosemary Roasted Chicken and Veggies

Total macros: Calories: 1,700, Fat: 128.5g, Protein: 103g, Net Carbs: 22g

Day 4

Breakfast: Lemon Poppy Ricotta Pancakes with 3 Slices Thick-Cut Bacon

Lunch: Leftover Spiced Pumpkin Soup with ½ Medium Avocado

Dinner: Leftover Rosemary Roasted Chicken and Veggies

Total macros: Calories: 1,665, Fat: 130g, Protein: 95.5g, Net Carbs: 23.5g

Day 5

Breakfast: Leftover Lemon Poppy Ricotta Pancakes with 3 Slices Thick-Cut Bacon

Lunch: Leftover Spiced Pumpkin Soup

Dinner: Cheesy Sausage Mushroom Skillet with 1

Slice Thick-Cut Bacon

Total macros: Calories: 1,650, Fat: 126g, Protein: 100.5g, Net Carbs: 22.5g

Day 6

Breakfast: Sweet Blueberry Coconut Porridge with 1 Slice Thick-Cut Bacon

Lunch: Leftover Easy Beef Curry

Dinner: Leftover Cheesy Sausage Mushroom Skillet

Total macros: Calories: 1,670, Fat: 112g, Protein: 100g, Net Carbs: 33.5g

Day 7

Breakfast: Leftover Sweet Blueberry Coconut Porridge

Lunch: Leftover Easy Beef Curry

Dinner: Lamb Chops with Rosemary and Garlic

Total macros: Calories: 1,625, Fat: 108g, Protein: 110.5g, Net Carbs: 27g

WEEK 2

Day 1

Breakfast: Fat-Busting Vanilla Protein Smoothie

Lunch: Easy Cheeseburger Salad

Dinner: Chicken Zoodle Alfredo

Total macros: Calories: 1,530, Fat: 113.5g, Protein: 107.5g, Net Carbs: 18.5g

Day 2

Breakfast: Savory Ham and Cheese Waffles with 2 Slices Thick-Cut Bacon

Lunch: Pan-Fried Pepperoni Pizzas

Dinner: Cabbage and Sausage Skillet

Total macros: Calories: 1,670, Fat: 129g, Protein: 103g, Net Carbs: 20.5g

Day 3

Breakfast: Mozzarella Veggie-Loaded Quiche with 1 Slice Thick-Cut Bacon

Lunch: Leftover Easy Cheeseburger Salad

Dinner: Gyro Salad with Avo-Tzatziki

Total macros: Calories: 1,580, Fat: 104.5g, Protein: 117.5g, Net Carbs: 33g

Day 4

Breakfast: Pepper Jack Sausage Egg Muffins with 3 Slices Thick-Cut Bacon

Lunch: Leftover Pan-Fried Pepperoni Pizza

Dinner: Leftover Cabbage and Sausage Skillet

Total macros: Calories: 1,650, Fat: 127.5g, Protein: 101g, Net Carbs: 29g

Day 5

Breakfast: Leftover Savory Ham and Cheese Waffles with 1 Slice Thick-Cut Bacon

Lunch: Leftover Cabbage and Sausage Skillet

Dinner: Leftover Chicken Zoodle Alfredo

Total macros: Calories: 1,620, Fat: 119g, Protein: 119g, Net Carbs: 18.5g

Day 6

Breakfast: Leftover Pepper Jack Sausage Egg Muffins with 1 Slice Thick-Cut Bacon

Lunch: Leftover Pan-Fried Pepperoni Pizza

Dinner: Leftover Gyro Salad with Avo-Tzatziki

Total macros: Calories: 1,595, Fat: 116g, Protein: 110g, Net Carbs: 15.5g

Day 7

Breakfast: Leftover Pepper Jack Sausage Egg Muffins with ½ Medium Avocado

Lunch: Leftover Cabbage and Sausage Skillet with 1 Slice Thick-Cut Bacon

Dinner: Leftover Gyro Salad with Avo-Tzatziki

Total macros: Calories: 1,605, Fat: 118.5g, Protein: 102g, Net Carbs: 22.5g

WEEK 3

Day 1

Breakfast: 3 Cloud Buns with 3 Tbsp. Peanut Butter and 3 Slices Thick-Cut Bacon

Lunch: Mozzarella Tuna Melt

Dinner: Cheesy Single-Serve Lasagna

Total macros: Calories: 1,605, Fat: 116.5g, Protein: 114.5g, Net Carbs: 28.5g

Day 2

Breakfast: Bacon Breakfast Bombs

Lunch: Avocado, Egg & Salami Sandwiches

Dinner: Crispy Chipotle Chicken Thighs

Total macros: Calories: 1,525, Fat: 118.5g, Protein: 99.5g, Net Carbs: 12g

Day 3

Breakfast: Three-Cheese Pizza Frittata with 3 Slices Thick-Cut Bacon

Lunch: Leftover Mozzarella Tuna Melt

Dinner: Pepperoni, Ham, and Cheddar Stromboli

Total macros: Calories: 1,660, Fat: 121g, Protein: 119g, Net Carbs: 22.5g

Day 4

Breakfast: 3 Cloud Buns with 3 Tbsp. Peanut Butter and 2 Slices Thick-Cut Bacon

Lunch: Leftover Three-Cheese Pizza Frittata with 2 Slices Thick-Cut Bacon

Dinner: Leftover Pepperoni, Ham, and Cheddar Stromboli

Total macros: Calories: 1,640, Fat: 130.5g, Protein: 100.5g, Net Carbs: 20.5g

Day 5

Breakfast: Leftover Bacon Breakfast Bombs

Lunch: Leftover Avocado, Egg & Salami Sandwiches with 1 Slice Thick-Cut Bacon

Dinner: Leftover Crispy Chipotle Chicken Thighs

Total macros: Calories: 1,625, Fat: 126.5g, Protein: 106.5g, Net Carbs: 12.5g

Day 6

Breakfast: Leftover Three-Cheese Pizza Frittata with 2 Slices Thick-Cut Bacon

Lunch: Leftover Pepperoni, Ham, and Cheddar Stromboli

Dinner: Spring Salad with Steak and Sweet Dressing

Total macros: Calories: 1,585, Fat: 120.5g, Protein: 108g, Net Carbs: 13.5g

Day 7

Breakfast: Leftover Three-Cheese Pizza Frittata with

2 Slices Thick-Cut Bacon

Lunch: Mushroom Soup with Fried Egg and 2 Slices Thick-Cut Bacon

Dinner: Leftover Spring Salad with Steak and Sweet Dressing

Total macros: Calories: 1,665, Fat: 130.5g, Protein: 110g, Net Carbs: 13.5g

WEEK 4

Day 1

Breakfast: Rocket Fuel Latte with Maca

Lunch: Zucchini Pasta Salad & Chicken

Dinner: *Carb Up* Flank Steak, Plantains & Watermelon Salad

Snack: Mojito Water

Day 2

Breakfast: Veggie Frittata

Lunch: Vanilla Creme Gummies

Dinner: Slaw with Chicken & Bacon

Snack: Tropical Coconut Balls

Day 3

Breakfast: Eggplant & Bacon Sauté

Lunch: Sardine Salad

Dinner: Chorizo Bowl

Snack: Jicama Fries

Day 4

Breakfast: Rocket Fuel Latte with Maca

Lunch: Zucchini Pasta Salad & Chicken

Dinner: *Carb Up* Flank Steak, Plantains & Watermelon Salad

Snack: Mojito Water

Day 5

Breakfast: Eggplant & Bacon Sauté

Lunch: Vanilla Creme Gummies

Dinner: Chorizo Bowl

Snack: Jicama Fries

Day 6

Breakfast: Veggie Frittata

Lunch: Sardine Salad

Dinner: Slaw with Chicken & Bacon

Snack: Tropical Coconut Balls

Day 7

Breakfast: Rocket Fuel Latte with Maca

Lunch: Zucchini Pasta Salad & Chicken

Dinner: *Carb Up* Flank Steak, Plantains & Watermelon Salad

Snack: Mojito Water

CHAPTER 6

THE KETO GROCERY LIST

The net carb content is listed next to each food.

Keto Nuts/Seeds

- (2 g per 1/4 cup) Almonds
- (1.4 g per tablespoon) Almond butter
- (2 g per 1/4 cup) Brazil nuts
- (4.1 g per 1/4 cup) Sunflower seeds
- (1.4 g per cup) Unsweetened almond milk
- (7 g per 1/4 cup) Cashews
- (4.4 g per tablespoon) Cashew butter
- (1 g per tablespoon) Chia seeds
- (0 g) Flax seeds
- (2 g per 1/4 cup) Hazelnuts
- (2 g per 3 tablespoons) Hemp seeds
- (2 g per 1/4 cup) Macadamia nuts
- (2 g per 1/4 cup) Pecans
- (3 g per 1/4 cup) Pine nuts
- (1 g per 1/4 cup) Pumpkin seeds
- (1.5 g per tablespoon) Sunflower butter
- (2 g per 1/4 cup) Walnuts

Keto Vegetables

- (2.4 g per cup) Asparagus
- (0.8 g per cup) Bok choy
- (3.6 g per cup) Broccoli
- (2 g per cup) Radishes
- (0.2 g per cup) Romaine lettuce
- (0.4 g per cup) Spinach
- (2.9 g per cup) Cabbage
- (3 g per cup) Cauliflower
- (1.6 g per cup) Celery
- (2.5 g per cup) Summer squash
- (0.8 g per cup) Swiss chard
- (2.4 g per cup) Zucchini
- (2 g per cup) Collard greens
- (1.9 g per cup) Cucumber
- (2.4 g per cup) Eggplant
- (1 g per cup) Iceberg lettuce
- (3.7 g per cup) Jalapeño peppers
- (0.1 g per cup) Kale
- (3.5 g per cup) Kohlrabi
- (1.6 g per cup) Mushrooms

Keto Pantry Items

- Avocado oil (0 g)
- Coconut butter (1 g per tablespoon)
- Coconut flour (3 g per 2 tablespoons)

- Coconut oil (0 g)
- Bone broth (0 g)
- Almond flour (1 g per 2 tablespoons)
- Erythritol (4 g per teaspoon)
- Ghee (0 g)
- Kelp noodles (2 g per 4 ounces)
- Mayonnaise (0.2 g per 2 tablespoons)
- MCT oil (0 g)
- Monk fruit extract (0 g)
- Olive oil (0 g)
- Canned full-fat coconut milk (3.6 g per 1/2 cup)
- Butter (0 g)
- Caesar dressing (0.4 g per tablespoon)
- Canola oil (0 g)
- Pesto (0.8 g per tablespoon)
- Ranch dressing (0.9 g per tablespoon)
- Sesame oil (0 g)
- Sugar-free chocolate (5 g per tablespoon)
- Stevia extract (3 g per teaspoon)
- Tahini (1.78 g per tablespoon)
- Walnut oil (0 g)
- Blue cheese dressing (0.7 g per tablespoon)

Keto Meat

- (0 g) Anchovies
- (0 g) Chicken wings

- (0 g) Ground beef
- (0 g) Sardines
- (0 g) Short ribs
- (0 g) Herring
- (0 g) Mackerel
- (1 g per 2 ounces) Pancetta
- (1.6 g per cup) Pepperoni
- (0 g) Pork belly
- (2.8 g per cup) Salami
- (0 g) Sardines
- (0 g) Bacon
- (3 g per 2 ounces) Sausage
- (0 g) Salmon
- (0 g) Porterhouse steak
- (0 g) Ribeye
- (0.02 g per 3 ounces) Chicken drumsticks or thighs

Keto Fruits

- (3.6 g per cup) Avocado
- (7.1 g per cup) Blackberries
- (17.8 g per cup) Blueberries
- (12.3 g per cup) Cantaloupe
- (5.4 g per fruit) Lemon
- (5.2 g per fruit) Lime
- (6.7 g per cup) Raspberries
- (8.2 g per cup) Strawberries

- (3.3 g per cup) Tomato
- (10.9 g per cup) Watermelon

Keto Eggs/Dairy

- (5.7 g per 1/2 cup) Unsweetened, full-fat yoghurt
- (5.3 g per 1/2 cup) Full-fat sour cream
- (5.9 per 1/2 cup) Whole milk
- (0 g) Eggs
- (1–3.8 g per ounce)Full-fat cheese
- (0.8 g per tablespoon) Full-fat cream cheese
- (4 g per 1/2 cup) Full-fat cottage cheese
- (2.5 g per 1/4 cup) Heavy whipping cream

To count on low-carb or keto diets, will you have calories?

When it comes to weight, calories are frequently talked about but are often mistaken. Yes, the fact that calorie counting is helpful in losing weight is debatable. Read on to learn about calories and their role in weight control in low-carb and keto diets.

CHAPTER 7
FAQ FOR KETO

H ere are some tips and tricks for common keto concerns, whether you're thinking about starting keto or you're five weeks in. Before making any major modifications to your diet, check with your doctor.

1. What foods am I supposed to eat on the KETO diet?

Stick to these principles for the best keto results:

An abundance of high-quality fats such as ghee and grass-fed butter, MCT oil, avocado oil, and coconut oil

Moderate amounts of fatty proteins, such as meat fed by grass, pastured eggs, fatty fish caught in the wild and protein from collagen.

Lots of low-carb and nutrient-dense vegetables, such as organic broccoli, zucchini, avocado, cucumbers, cabbage and celery.

Check out this downloadable complete keto food list

for a more detailed guide on what to eat on the keto diet.

2. If I'm in Ketosis, how do I know?

Depending on your body's ability to adapt to burning fat for fuel, it can take anywhere from 2-3 days to a few weeks to get into ketosis. Your body will naturally produce ketones once you get into ketosis, molecules that fuel your brain and body with fat, not carbs.

If you have steady, lasting energy, better focus, and a reduced appetite, you can usually tell if you are in ketosis. Test your blood ketone levels for definitive answers. When your ketone levels measure 0.5-3, you are in ketosis (that's millimoles per litre).

Using urine sticks, blood sticks or a blood meter, you can test your levels. Using a breath analyser, you can also test for acetone levels in your breath.

Just tracking how your body feels, though it is an easy way to know if you've hit that sweet spot of ketosis. Here are indications that you may be in ketosis:

Reduced hunger: your hunger hormones are suppressed by ketones, helping you feel fuller longer.

Keto breath: Because of raised ketone levels, people

often experience a metallic taste in their mouth.

Weight loss: The keto diet burns fat, so you're likely to get ketosis if you lose weight.

Flu-like symptoms: You may experience keto flu symptoms such as headaches, chills and lightheadedness when you first start.

3. Do I need macros to be calculated, and how do I count them?

The carbs, fats and protein that make up your food and help you create energy are macros or macronutrients. Counting macros on the keto diet isn't essential, but it's a useful way to learn more about your food and understand the needs of your body. Learn more about ideal keto macros, including the advantages of counting them (and disadvantages).

4. Do I need net carbs to be calculated?

You should keep track of net carbs, even if you don't calculate macros, the carbs that your body uses for energy. Net carbohydrate calculation can help you to remain in ketosis and inform your food choices. Find out how to calculate net keto carbs and how many net carbs you need vs total carbs.

5. Are KETO diets healthy?

The ketogenic diet is reliable and supported by science. The keto diet has been shown to support weight loss, create more mitochondria in your brain and decrease inflammation when done properly.

However, depending on what you put on your plate, any diet can be good or bad for you. When you stick to the Bulletproof Diet roadmap, you eliminate keto foods such as processed cheese and sugar-free sodas that make you feel weak and do not belong to a healthy diet.

6. ABOUT "DIRTY KETO? "

Dirty keto follows the standard keto diet's same high-fat low-carb structure, but it allows for processed packaged and fast foods. While you're on dirty keto, you can still get into ketosis and burn fat, but it has serious drawbacks like inflammation and weight gain. Here are the dirty keto facts, and why you should avoid them.

8. Does the KETO diet cause DIABETES?

No, diabetes is not caused by Keto. Several studies indicate that by reducing glucose intolerance and stabilizing blood sugar, ketosis may help manage diabetes.

9. Is the long-term KETO DIET sustainable?

Yeah, yes and no. Some individuals thrive without any problems on the full keto diet. Other individuals face long-term carbohydrate restriction problems, such as insomnia and hormone imbalances. If this is the case, experiment with cycling with keto carb (aka cyclic ketosis) where one day a week you eat a moderate amount of carbohydrates, so that your body can cycle in and out of ketosis. It is an efficient change that helps many individuals avoid any potential dangers and hazards of a keto diet. Here's how, and whether it's right for you, to do a keto carb cycling diet. It is always a good idea to review your diet frequently with your doctor.

10. What are the various types of ketones?

Three kinds of ketone bodies exist. They are:

- Acetoacetate (AcAc): This is the first type of ketone made from fatty acids by your body.

- Beta-hydroxybutyric acid (BHB): The

transformation of acetoacetate into beta-hydroxybutyric acid. BHB, based on its chemical structure, is not a ketone, but it is still considered part of the ketone family because it works similarly to others. Fun fact: Brain Octane oil is a BHB precursor, a purified form of MCT oil.

- Acetone: Acetone is the least abundant ketone in the blood, a by-product of acetoacetate. It passes through the breath or urine of the body.

You'll produce more of each type the longer you fast or restrict carbs.

11. If I need more CARBS, how do I know?

Some individuals feel fine for extended periods when they eat very few carbs. But your body may be asking for more carbs if you are dealing with symptoms such as dry eyes, insomnia, fatigue and mood swings, especially if you are a woman, an athlete or dealing with a lot of stress (or all of the above). Learn more about the benefits of using your carb intake to experiment.

12. Why am I not losing weight with KETO?

You might be eating too much, not enough or

completely the wrong foods. Here are a few reasons why you don't lose weight on keto and what you should do about it.

13.   How is MCT OIL working with KETO?

In the ketogenic diet, MCT oil is a powerful tool because it helps your body produce more ketones and stay in ketosis. Not all MCT oils are the same, however, and some are more efficient than others. Here are the MCT oil and keto guide.

14. Should I Take Exogenous Ketones? Should I?

Exogenous ketones are synthetic ketones that help your blood to increase ketone levels. They're popular supplements, but not required — instead, focus on eating enough high-quality fats. Your body will naturally produce all the ketones you need to power through your day. MCT oil is a great place to start if you want to add a supplement to your keto diet. Here you can read about the efficiency of various keto supplements.

15. Should I try INTERMITTENT FASTING ON KETO?

Definitely. Surely. By boosting your fat-burning and weight loss outcomes, intermittent fasting can make keto more effective. Learn more about intermittent fasting and keto fasting.

16. Is KETO the same as the diet of Atkins?

Hey, no. A keto diet contains moderate amounts of protein, whereas the Atkins Diet is extremely high in protein. On a keto diet, in a process called gluconeogenesis, large amounts of protein can turn into glucose, thus taking you out of ketosis. This is why fatty meat cuts are better than a chicken breast, which is high in protein and low in fat.

17. KETOGENIC DIET VS STANDARD KETO: WHAT'S THE DIFFERENCE?

You time your carb intake around workouts or times of heavy stress with targeted keto, to give your body a little extra fuel. During intense workouts, many people on a full keto diet report "bonking": They suddenly run out of fuel and don't have the energy to keep going. Research indicates that you are likely to run out of energy during anaerobic workouts with full keto, any kind of short, intense workout. That includes lifting, CrossFit and training for high-intensity intervals.

In the meantime, full keto, like long runs, seems to be good for endurance training. These are super-athletes, however, who are used to running up to 200 miles at a time. If you do not fit that bill, before a longer cardio session, you may benefit from doing targeted keto and having some carbs.

The other benefit is metabolic flexibility for targeted keto. People who stay long-term in ketosis gradually lose their ability to process carbs and can develop insulin resistance. That's fine as long as you never eat carbs. Still, with a targeted keto diet or a cyclical keto diet, you're better off breaking ketosis occasionally if you want to have maximum metabolic flexibility.

With the targeted ketogenic diet, the trick is to consume just enough carbs. During your workout, you want to burn through them and return to ketosis a few hours after exercise.

When you want higher-glycemic carbs, this is one of the rare times. During your workout, your goal is to burn through them for quick energy and have them out of your system by the time you finish. With that in mind, a few good carbohydrate options are:

- White rice

- Cassava

- Sweet potato baked

- Beets (as a bonus, you will get a nitric oxide boost, which gives more oxygen to your muscles)

- White potato (if you tolerate nightshades)

Note: you do not want to eat high-fructose keto-targeted carbohydrates. Instead of your muscles, fructose goes straight to your liver, so you'll end up dropping out of ketosis without offering extra energy to your muscles. Fruit, honey and agave are included in higher-fructose carbs. Steer clear of the keto-targeted ones.

Drizzle Brain Octane MCT oil on your pre-workout carb source for the ultimate boost, so that you have ketones for maximum energy and metabolic flexibility alongside the carbs.

CHAPTER 8
TIPS & TRICKS FOR KETO DIET

The 15 best keto diet tips and tricks to start and stick to! This list includes tips for keto success, simple keto recipes and beginner meal plans, and more when you're searching for keto details for beginners.

1. START EASY

Keep it straightforward, especially at the start. The easiest way to start keto is for beginners to use a basic structure for their meals:

1. Choose foods like chicken, beef, pork, turkey, shrimp, seafood, powdered protein, eggs, etc.

2. Choose a low-carb veggie: cauliflower, broccoli, zucchini, Brussels sprouts, cucumbers, bell peppers, etc.

3. Add a little fat. Butter, lard, sugar, ghee, milk, bacon, avocado, hemp, nuts, etc.

2. THE TEMPTATIONS BLOCK.

Some of the best tips for following a keto diet is to

get rid of things you need to stop. Sticking to your goals is much easier if you are not always dealing with the urge. Get rid of the following items in your fridge and countertop:

- Grains such as wheat, bread, pasta, rice, beans and corn, etc.

- Sugar table, sweets, pastries, biscuits, ice cream, coffee, soda, water, tea, maple syrup, etc.

- Starchy vegetables such as parsnips, onions, and sweet potatoes etc.

- Beans, lentils, chickpeas, and so on include legumes (The peanuts are a mild exception)

- Sugar-rich fruits, including bananas, pineapples, oranges, strawberries, grapes and so on.

- As with all cow's milk (except fine heavy cream), low-fat cheese and so on, low-fat meat & milk.

- In particular, margarine seed & vegetable oils, canola oil, corn oil, grape seed oil and soybean oil,

Read the label for hidden sugar, starch and chemical

ingredients, processed 'low carb' foods based on ingredients,

It can't be possible to get rid of anything if your family is not on board with low carb eating, and that's great!

Buy and store anything that you want to avoid when others in your family want to start consuming these items, so you can at least avoid a certain cupboard, refrigerator shelf, etc.

3. STOCK YOUR FRIDGE.

In addition to getting rid of all the wrong things, fill your fridge with lots of good things:

- Healthy fats, such as avocado oil, coconut oil and butter

- Leafy greens, such as lettuce, spinach, and kale

- Low carbonated vegetables that grow above ground, such as zucchini, cauliflower and asparagus

- Food for beef and pork

- Fowl with chicken and turkey

- Seafood such as cod and tuna

- Full-fat cheese and cheese high in cream

- Eggs Eggs

- Low carb fruits such as avocados, raspberries and coconuts (an exception to fruits that need not be moderate).

4. STOCK YOUR PANTRY

Do not forget to store in stock your keto staples too! It is most likely that pantry items are high in carbohydrates, so here are the types of products you would like to keep:

Cinnamon, basil and dill such as herbs & spices

High carbonated condiments such as mayo, mustard, and chilli sauce

Nuts & almond seeds, sunflower seeds, macadamia nuts and

Sugar-free sweeteners such as erythritol, monkey fruit and allulose;

Strong carbide flours such as almond meal, flaxseed meal and coconut meal

Sugar-free drinks, such as wine, coffee and tea

Alzheimer's disease: a ketogenic diet might improve Alzheimer's patients.

Cancer: Some studies indicate that in cancer therapy, ketogenic diets can be successful, possibly by helping glucose cells "starve."

Parkinson's disease: A small study revealed that after 28 days on the ketogenic diet, Parkinson's symptoms improved.

Acne: There is some evidence that this diet may reduce acne incidence and growth.

5. EASE INTO IT

Cold turkey can be a surprise if you start a keto diet that comes from consuming lots of carbs and sugar, taking all of it out. This can trigger (temporary) keto flu symptoms and cravings, and while these can be manageable, it does not mean that this is the only way to do so.

Here are several ways that can help ease it:

Apply a few of these keto tips and tricks at once,

leaving you time for improvements to be made.

Take out your food little by little. Then eliminate all fats, such as candy and soda, then complex carbohydrates, such as pasta and bread, and finally starchy veggies and berries.

Listen and be careful of your body. Try drinking some water, brushing your teeth, distracting yourself with something fun to do or just waiting for your brain to catch up for 20 minutes when you've finished your meal and are still hungry. After that, try a salty, water-packed snack, like olives or pickles, if you are still hungry.

6. PROTEIN ARE A LIMIT IS A GOAL & FAT IS A LEVER.

The most important key to going through ketosis is limiting carbohydrates, but there is more to it. A role is played by all the other macros, short for macronutrients.

In short, for a keto diet, here's how macros should be interpreted:

ARE CARBS A LIMIT.

For most people, it means that you set the amount

you will eat every day, usually up to 20 to 30 grams a day. If you go under that number, it's okay then! This is not a hard target; it's just a cap.

PROTEIN IS A GOAL.

Which implies that every day you want to reach this number, so try not to go under the mark. Going over a little bit is also okay, but a large amount of protein will turn to glucose and kick you out of ketosis; it varies from person to person how quickly this happens.

FAT IS A LEVER

The rest of the calories you need for the day come from fat, after your carb limit and protein target. This is what makes you satisfied and gives the bulk of your supply of energy.

Depending on your goals, you can use fat as a lever, raising it up or down. If you're hungry, raise it, minimize it to weight loss, but remember that you can't go too far (do not get caught in the old fat is evil" trap) because it's your primary energy source.

How do I define my macros?

So how do you know the numbers for the above

concepts that you can use? In our macro keto calculator, just enter your info.

DO NEED More FIBER?

It's more of a discussion here. USDA guidelines say 25-31 grams per day and 25-38 grams per day are recommended.

Several studies suggest that eating more fibre reduces the risk of heart disease and cancer, but fibre rates have been lower than the guidelines (14-26 grams per day of 25-38). You should eat much less than the "official" suggestions.

Start with 15-20 grams of fibre a day and, depending on how you feel, add more than a few grams at a time if necessary. Get as much fibre as possible from whole foods until using a supplement (vegetables, nuts, etc.)

KNOWING IF MY MACROS ARE CORRECT?

If the results you see for your macros are right, you'll know.

As some community members have said, "measure, measure, measure" and take photos. The scale alone does not rely on them. You will also see a difference in how your clothes fit, or the body's measurements before the scale catches up.

If you don't see any improvements after a few weeks, make sure you're truly in ketosis first and don't get any carbohydrates that sneak in. If you are, look at the fat lever and see if you can nudge it down.

7. PORTIONS DO MATTER

Portions are about the keto above tip #6 for diet. Although the primary focus of a ketogenic lifestyle is not calories and portions, they are still important.

On keto, you will still not lose weight or even add weight if you eat too much-this will be the case for any diet. The thing to bear in mind is that a lever is a fat.

Luckily, ketosis decreases appetite and cravings naturally, and you want to consume less anyway. Most individuals think that consuming low-carb foods automatically keeps their portions under control, but you may need to pay attention to them if that does not happen to you.

8. EAT whenever needed.

When you're not hungry, one common question I get

is whether you can eat. Ketosis acts as a natural appetite suppressant, so you may find that you don't get hungry as often or ravenously as you do.

There is no need to eat when you are not hungry! Only focus when you're hungry and sleeping on reaching your protein target, but then let your body signal when you're sleeping.

9. THE FLU-KETO AVOID.

You may have heard of keto fever, or maybe you have just had side effects with keto-start. It is one of the most popular questions on the keto diet for beginners.

As your body shifts its primary source of fuel from glucose and carbohydrates to ketones and fat, it will take your body some time to adapt to this metabolic transition. In the body, even ketosis flushes a lot of water that can cause the levels of electrolytes to drop.

How to prevent KETO FLU?

The good news is that and can be prevented; keto influenza is acute.

To prevent keto flu, make sure you get enough electrolytes to avoid (especially sodium, potassium and magnesium). Salting your food generously is one of the best things you can do here; some individuals even add sea salt to their water. It can also help to slowly ease it in.

FREQUENT HEADACHES ON KETO?

It is most likely to be due to either dehydration or depletion of electrolytes, which may be a mild type of keto flu. You should manage it the same way, with water and electrolytes.

10. REMAIN HYDRATED

Drinking water is great for everyone but especially if you're into ketosis. Eating carbohydrates enables us to retain more water in our bodies, while a keto diet flushes out more water, so it is even more important to consume enough. Aim at getting 16 cups a day.

11. MAKE RECIPES FOR KETO.

Keto recipes don't have to adhere 100 % to a keto lifestyle, but they make things easier and more enjoyable! For a long time to come, it will help you stick to it by getting the basics down, adding your old comfort food recipes in keto forms, such as keto bread or keto casseroles.

CONCLUSION

O besity is one of the world's known health issues. Several similar disorders are associated with it, ·collectively known as metabolic syndrome. These include high blood pressure, high blood sugar and a poor lipid profile in the blood.

There is a much greater risk of heart disease and type 2 diabetes for people with metabolic syndrome than for someone whose weight is in the normal range.

Much research has centred over the past decades on the causes of obesity and how it could be avoided or treated. Many individuals tend to believe that a lack of willpower triggers weight gain and obesity. That isn't completely true. While weight gain is largely a result of eating behaviour and lifestyle, when it comes to regulating their eating habits, some people are at a disadvantage.

The thing is, different biological factors such as ¬netics and hormones are driven by overeating. Some individuals are predisposed to weight gain. Of course, by modifying their lifestyle and behaviour, individuals can overcome their genetic disadvantages. Changes in lifestyles require willpower, commitment and perseverance. Nevertheless, it is much too simplistic to say that action is solely a feature of willpower. They do not take all the other factors into account that ultimately determine what individuals do and when they do it.

The storage of eggs in the ovary declines as women get older, and their ability to conceive decreases. Less oestrogen is released at this time, causing the body to behave differently. However, overnight, the body does not stop processing oestrogen, and the process may even take several years, during which symptoms gradually occur. The 'peri-menopause' is named this incremental adjustment.

The menstrual cycle ends fully at about the age of 50-55 years, so no more ovulations, no more cycles and no more pregnancies. That's the menopause here.

This loss of reproductive capacity can be profoundly felt in some women, and menopause is a personal experience for all women, not just a medical disorder.

Menopause hormonal changes will make you more likely than around your hips and thighs to gain weight around your belly. Yet hormonal shifts alone don't usually result in weight gain from menopause. Instead, weight gain, as well as lifestyle and genetic factors, are typically linked to ageing.

For instance, with age, muscle mass usually decreases, while fat increases. Losing muscle mass slows the pace at which calories are utilized by your body (metabolism). This can make keeping a healthy weight more difficult. You're likely to gain weight if you continue eating as you always have and don't increase your physical activity.

CPSIA information can be obtained
at www.ICGtesting.com
Printed in the USA
LVHW010510220221
679516LV00003B/179

9 781801 766067